W9-AKY-264

Healing with HERBS

Nature's Way to Better Health

Henrietta A. Diers Rau

**ARCO PUBLISHING, INC.
NEW YORK**

Dedicated to my husband

for

his patience and encouragement

Published by Arco Publishing, Inc.
219 Park Avenue South, New York, N.Y. 10003
by arrangement with Pageant Poseidon Press Ltd.

Previously published under the title *Nature's Aid*.

Copyright © 1968 by Henrietta A. Diers Rau

All rights reserved. No part of this book may be
reproduced by any means or in any form without
permission in writing from the publisher,
except by a reviewer.

Library of Congress Catalog Card Number 75-23579
ISBN 0-668-03878-0

Printed in the United States of America

10 9 8 7 6

CONTENTS

PREFACE

WHY HAVE I written this book? I have been asked this question many times. It has been a lot of work and many years in the making, but I did have a purpose in mind which kept me digging for more and more information.

I had been interested in healing herbs many years before my beloved mother and only sister were stricken with cancer. Told time and again that there was no hope for them, I turned to the information that I had already gathered. I feel that I did make their "waiting" time less painful and oh, how I wished then that I knew more.

When my mother could keep nothing in her stomach, I gave her red elm gruel, which stayed down, and she enjoyed it too. When she could not swallow, I fed her red elm gruel with an eye dropper. Later we progressed to baby bottles. I bought an automatic baby bottle warmer and kept a supply of bottles on hand for her when she was hungry. I crushed vitamin tablets into the gruel for added nutrition.

Being confined to bed, Mother had bowel compaction. The customary soap enema made her sick for three or four days. I learned to give her an olive oil enema, and she was relieved quickly and easily.

I purchased a juicer and gave my mother and sister raw carrots and other vegetable juices; also grape juice.

We use dandelion, peppermint, spearmint, violet, and chickweed leaves from our garden for tea and salad. Chickweed I also made into an ointment. Plantain and grape leaves from our garden are our favorite leaves as a poultice for all kinds of sores. Try them the next time you burn yourself. You will be surprised at the results. You do not run to the doctor with a common

1

burn, but it can be painful. In the winter, we use sea onion, which has been transferred to the house.

I must tell you about my experience with grape leaves. We were in the country 8 miles from a doctor when I fell through the porch floor and was wedged in right up to my thigh. My husband had to saw through the attached boards to release me. I was badly bruised. My husband wanted to take me to the doctor, but I asked him to get wild grape leaves and to wrap my entire leg with them. In 2 days you would not know that I had been injured except for a few small spots that were still black and blue. I had no pain at all. We use grape leaves for many sores, especially burns. They heal very quickly and with a minimum of pain. I could mention many other instances.

In Greece and some other countries they use grape leaves in their cooking and for wrapping food. They seem to know the values of these leaves.

However, if you need the services of a medical doctor, by all means do not neglect to see one.

I have studied and researched medical herbs now for a number of years, receiving my diploma as Master of Herbalism from Dominion Herbal College, Ltd. of Canada and Diploma of Naturopathy from the Anglo-American Institute of Drugless Therapy in England.

People are again becoming interested in this ancient form of the healing arts, as evidenced by the increasing demands for these remedies at the herb stores.

My husband and I (we are senior citizens) enjoy going into the country to search for the various plants, to recognize them, and to study their healing qualities. This hobby has been a source of conversation, and we are always amazed at the interest that people display.

This is the reason I have made up a book of the information I have gathered over many years.

HENRIETTA A. DIERS RAU

Rahway, N.J.

NATURE'S AID

PREVENTION *is the cry of today: prevent war, prevent fire, prevent ghettos and slums, prevent unemployment, and prevent the insecurity of old age. All of these are receiving their share of publicity, except PREVENT ILLNESS. This shall, therefore, be our aim.*

PREVENTION IS BETTER THAN A CURE

FIRST OF ALL, if there is any question about your health, consult a medical doctor; he is trained for that purpose.

This book is to acquaint you with the possibilities in plants known to you as vegetables, condiments, spices, and herbs. These and their present uses may be familiar to you, but you may not know the way these were used in former years; years when people depended on knowledge of plant uses handed down from generation to generation. I read in the papers that researchers are digging into the botanists' file for new, old plants to add to their list of drugs. Why can't we make use of these plants before they are synthesized and put on the drugstore shelves? I am told the reason is that the plants work slower in the body than the synthesized parts. EZEKIEL 47:12—"The fruit thereof shall be for meat and the leaf for medicine." PSALM 104:14—"He causeth the grass to grow for the cattle and herb for the service of man." ROMANS 14:2—"For one believeth that he may eat all things; another, who is weak, eateth herbs." The whole plant,

3

according to the Bible, is NATURE'S AID for your most precious possession, YOUR HEALTH.

A commentator on the radio one evening a short time ago remarked that doctors do not cure disease; they ASSIST the body to cure itself. These same doctors spend ten years training to recognize the disease to which the body is host. Most doctors, today, are specializing, and the general practitioner is becoming more scarce every day. So is hospital space.

The American Indian, or our forefather, did not have the services of such doctors or the efficient hospital and staff to which we have become accustomed.

So why not practice a little PREVENTION and perhaps give our harried doctors a break?

Time was when vegetables, as we know them today, were grown in the wild state—many still do. These vegetables, or plants, contain all the life-saving ingredients, if we would but use them for our benefit. Every health need of the human body is found in plants. In fact herbal healing is the most ancient form of healing known. No matter how far back we look in history, man sought a remedy for his ailments in the fields and woods with remarkable success.

Among the ancient Jews, the priests were the healers, and it is generally accepted that the tithes of thyme, mint, and other herbs (as mentioned in the Bible) were their *materia medica*.

The Egyptians, 3500 years ago before Christ, well knew the uses of myrrh, turpentine, olive oil, cummin, cassia, peppermint, caraway seed, juniper berries, etc.

Hippocrates, called the Father of Medicine, depended on the use of herbs for his success.

The African and the North American Indian, in their native states, wrought cures with simple herbs.

In Old England, the girls in the family were taken out to the fields by their parents and taught the names and the healing virtues of the plants. This was the start of their popular herb gardens.

Today herbal healing is a lost art. As we look at the records, no one can deny that with all the wonder drugs on the market, there is a constant demand for more doctors, more nurses, and more hospitals.

Why not take a candid look at the present health situation

4

and try a little PREVENTION through the use of Herbs? ISAIAH 40:7—"All flesh is grass and all the goodliness thereof is as the flower of the field."

Living man is a vital organism with a vital force resident in the bioplasm of the cell, the only acting force in health or disease. It is the bioplasm which selects, disintegrates, assimilates, and converts to its own use the therapeutic value of any remedial agent used.

Vital force draws all its material from one source, the blood, for "The Blood is the Life." From this source, each cell takes what it needs, and out of this is fashioned brain, muscle, skin, tendon, bone, and hair. Herbs have in them inherent properties which the vital force can use in an effort to restore the body to normal.

A good slogan could be "Keep your Blood free of impurities."

I have just finished reading a book written for children by an M.D. in 1872. In it he explains the relationship between plants and humans. I think you will find it as interesting and informative as I did. The following is a brief resume:

The root is the STOMACH of the plant. It has many little MOUTHS in its branches everywhere that suck up the food, a fluid, from the ground. This fluid is the sap that goes up in the stalk to nourish the plant. Everything in the plant, the bark, the wood, the leaves, the flowers, and the fruit is made from this sap and also the root.

The plants never make a mistake about the food they choose. We sometimes make mistakes about our food.

The sap goes up one set of pipes to the leaves and down to the roots through another set of pipes, just as our blood (sap) circulates by going into the arteries (pipes) from the heart and back to the heart through the veins (pipes). As in our circulation, the sap (blood) is not a perfect sap as it goes to the leaves (our lungs), which have breathing pores (respiration), for an airing before it is of any use. It then goes down to the very roots and up to the leaves again. It is this aired sap (blood) which makes every part of the plant (body) grow. The chief use of our breathing is to air the blood.

The blood, then, is to your body what the sap is to the plant, the building material. Out of the blood is made the skin, the hair, the nails, the soft red gums, the hard white teeth in the mouth, the complex eye, and the parts inside that you cannot see, such as the hard bones, the red muscles, the cords, the light spongy lungs, the thick firm liver, the soft brain, the nerves, the digesting machinery, etc. And that is not all. The wax in your ears, the bile, the tears, the arteries, the veins in which the blood runs, and even the heart that pumps the blood is itself made from the blood. This applies to all parts of the body.

The plants get the food out of the earth for us and put it into such a shape that our stomachs can use it. We may say that the plant's stomach gathers food out of the ground for our stomachs.

The same thing is true when you eat meat. This meat was once a part of the ground.

There is a reason for the expression Mother Earth, as the earth is our mother in the sense that we get all our food from it.

Some plants are sugar factories, some are gum factories, some are starch factories, some are perfume factories, some are color factories, and some plants are MEDICINE FACTORIES.

HERBS

Part I

HERBS

The herbs here listed are well-known and can be used to perform specific tasks. Some of these can be combined, if necessary.

The general methods of preparing herbs are by infusion, decoction, or extraction.

An infusion is made by steeping one teaspoonful of leaves or flowers in one cup of boiling water for 5 to 10 minutes.

A decoction is made by boiling the roots and/or seeds in water for 15 to 20 minutes.

The usual dose of either infusion or decoction is one or 2 cups taken daily, sipped slowly.

The extract is prepared by a chemist (or pharmacist), and his directions should be followed.

MEASURES CALLED FOR:

1 t.—1 teaspoonful
1 T.—1 Tablespoonful
1 C.—1 Cup
F.E.—Fluid Extract
Elix.—Elixir

APOTHECARIES' LIQUID MEASURE

60 minims	—1 fl. dram
8 fluid drams	—1 fl. oz.
16 ″ oz.	—1 pt.
8 pts.	—1 gal.
3 or 4 T.	—1 Wine glassful

20 grains	—1 scruple
3 scruples	—1 dram
8 drams	—1 oz.
12 oz.	—1# approx.

PRICKLY ASH (*Xanthoxylum Fraxineum*)

Prickly ash is a native of Northern, Middle, and Western America. It should not be confused with the Southern prickly ash, properly called angelica tree (*Aralia Spinosa*).

The LEAVES and the CAPSULES have an aromatic odor resembling oil of lemon. The BARK is the official portion, boiling water and alcohol extract its medical virtues.

Chewing the bark is said to relieve toothaches, and, because of this, it is often called the "toothache tree." The taste is warm, aromatic, and slightly bitter.

Prickly ash BARK induces a good, free capillary and arterial circulation, stimulates the stomach, the lymphatics, the serous and mucous membranes and, when chewed, the salivary glands, inducing a free flow of saliva. It is valuable wherever a stimulant is required, as when the skin and extremities are cold, and in many chronic conditions such as rheumatism, neuralgia, and paralysis.

It enjoys a considerable reputation as a remedy for chronic rheumatism. The dose of the powder is from 10 grains to ½ drachm. to be repeated 3 or 4 times daily. Or a decoction may be prepared by boiling an ounce of prickly ash bark in 3 pints of water down to 1 quart. One pint may be taken in divided doses during 24 hours.

A good formula for rheumatism is as follows: prickly ash bark ½ oz., bogbean and guaiacum chips each ½ oz., cayenne ⅛ t. Boil in 1½ pints water for 15 minutes. Strain and take a wine-glassful 3 or 4 times daily.

If the hands and feet are cold as the result of a sluggish circulation, take a simple infusion of 1 t. bark in 1 C. boiling water, drinking 1 C. daily.

The powdered bark applied externally cleans and stimulates old wounds and indolent ulcers to a healthy tone.

The SEEDS or BERRIES are considered slightly more stimulating than the bark.

The OIL is considered the best. Fill a bottle full of the berries and add non-poisonous alcohol. Allow to stand a week or more. Evaporate the alcohol and you have the oil.

Prickly ash acts slower than capsicum, but its effects are more permanent when taken in small and frequent doses.

Prickly ash bark is thought to resemble mezereum and guaiacum in its remedial action, and is taken for the same complaints.

BALM OF GILEAD (Populus Balsamifera)

This tree is also known as the Carolina poplar and is used as a shade tree. The BUDS are gathered in the spring before they expand. They are balsamic, somewhat sticky, and exude a resinous substance of a fragrant odor, which, in medicinal properties, somewhat resembles the gum myrrh, with a bitterish, balsamic, and somewhat pungent taste. These buds must be soaked in alcohol to dissolve the resin before they can be used in an infusion, as water alone does not extract all their virtues.

While chiefly influencing the respiratory organs, they are slightly stimulating to the circulation. They have quite a reputation in helping old, long standing coughs, dry asthma, and pulmonic debility. They should NOT BE USED, however, in recent inflammatory conditions.

A useful tincture is made by bruising 2 oz. of the buds and steeping them in 1 quart of medicinal alcohol. This can be added to cough syrups, and is also good for bathing sores.

An excellent healing ointment is made by boiling the buds in olive oil or leaf lard.

Balm of Gilead is considered the proper turpentine and of greater excellence for sores and ulcers.

The *Bible Dictionary* says of balm of Gilead: "An odoriferous resin, highly esteemed in the East for its healing virtues. It was an article of commerce between the Jews and the Tyrians."

BALMONY (Chelone Glabra)

Balmony, a native of North America, grows in the damp soils all over the U.S.

Its virtues are imparted to water or alcohol.

Where a torpid liver is involved, balmony is one of our finest

11

tonics. By its influence, it arouses gastric and salivary secretions, and by its effect upon the biliary and fecal discharges and in cleansing the system of morbid secretions of bile, the whole assimilating organism is toned up, stimulating the appetite and toning the stomach. It may be freely used in atonic conditions. In dyspepsia, debility, chronic jaundice, and constipation, it is very useful. Where there is much depression, add balmony to alteratives.

Combine with butternut in cases of constipation for better results. In dropsical conditions, with chronic hepatic and gastric torpor, combined with diuretics, the tonic properties of balmony will be extended in the direction of the kidneys.

Balmony has long been considered a certain remedy for worms in children and for stomach worms. An infusion of 1 oz. to 1 pint boiling water can be taken freely in wine-glass doses.

For irritated and itching piles, use an ointment made from fresh balmony leaves.

BARBERRY (Berberis Vulgaris)

This shrub is found throughout most of the U.S.

The BERRIES are a pleasant acidulous fruit, cooling and refreshing as a drink in acute diseases. They are also used in making pies and jams.

The BARK of the stem infused in beer is said to be useful in jaundice. The dose is from 1 to 2 oz. twice daily.

As a corrector of secretions of the liver it is possibly without equal. Its influence upon the liver is such that the bile will flow more freely, making it useful in practically all liver troubles, bilious conditions, and jaundice. Wherever the bile has been absorbed, upsetting the digestion and tinging the skin, use barberry. It is useful in fevers, loss of appetite, spleen affections, and will assist in constipation. It expels and removes morbid matter from the stomach and bowels.

It is because of these properties that it was much used by some patent medicine vendors. Many years ago, in New England, a tincture was made by steeping the bark in hard cider. It was made as follows:

Barberry, white poplar, and wild cherry barks, each 4 oz. These were crushed and steeped 1 week in a gallon of cider, strained, and a dose of 1 T. or more taken 3 times daily. This would have quite a tonic effect on the digestive tract and would be useful in biliousness, particularly debilitated cases, and in convalescence.

Because of its antiseptic properties, a decoction of the bark or berries will make an excellent gargle or mouth-wash.

Barberry may be used in infusion, decoction, tincture, fluid extract, solid extract, pills, capsules, powder, or syrup.

The bark dyes a beautiful yellow.

BAYBERRY (Myrica Cerifera)

Bayberry is an aromatic shrub growing over most of the U.S. It is considered by many to be one of the most useful and valuable herbs in the botanic field.

The fruit, or BERRIES, are covered with a whitish coating of wax which is separated for use. This vegetable wax is sometimes substituted for bees wax in the formation of plasters. The name "candleberry" was given to it because it was used in the making of tapers and candles. It is somewhat fragrant, when burning, but emits a less brilliant light than common lamp oil.

The process of collecting the wax is simple. The berries are boiled in water, the wax melting and floating on the surface, or allowed to concrete as it cools, is removed in the solid state. To render it pure, it is again melted and strained. It has a feeble odor and a slightly bitterish taste.

This wax possesses mild astringent properties, and has been popularly employed as a remedy for diarrhea and dysentery, and we are told it was found to be of great advantage during an epidemic of this complaint. The powdered wax was mixed with a syrup and taken in doses of 1 t., frequently repeated.

The OIL distilled from the BERRIES is used in bay rum as a hair dressing.

The BARK of the root is the official part. It should be collected in the latter part of the fall. When thoroughly dry, pulverize and keep in a closed container. Water is employed to extract the astringent principles and alcohol to extract its stimulating properties. The taste is astringent, bitter, and pungent. The odor is slightly aromatic.

Its stimulating properties arouse the whole circulation. If combined with a little capsicum in a warm infusion, it will improve arterial and capillary circulation and tone up the tissues.

As an astringent, it will not dry the mucus membrane but will promote glandular activity and restore the mucous secretions to a normal activity.

In sore throat, especially a putrid sore throat, gargle with an infusion of 1 t. to 1 pint boiling water. It will clean the mucous membrane of all morbid matter. After the gargle, a drink of the infusion will clean the most vile matter out of the stomach in 3 minutes. The infusion is also a good wash for ulcers and for spongy and bleeding gums.

Large doses may induce nausea and vomiting. Its promptness in this respect, however, has caused it to be used with success in narcotic poisoning and mercurial cachexia. If the poison is still in the stomach after a strong, hot infusion of bayberry, follow up with a lobelia emetic, and the poison will be expelled by vomiting.

In hemorrhage of the uterus, bowels, lungs, Leucorrhea, and in excessive menstruation, an infusion of bayberry is most valuable. It is recommended in prolapsus uteri, and in partuition it will be directly manifest in firmer contractions and will check possible flooding. Its influence on the uterus is very positive.

In goitre, good results have been had from doses of 10 gr. of the powder 3 times daily.

In buboes, carbuncles, scrofulous ulcers, gangrenous sores, etc., apply the powder as a poultice.

In adenoids, nasal congestion or catarrh, the powder, as a snuff, will give fine results. Dip one end of a straw in the powder, placing the other end in the nostril, and have someone blow the powder in or snuff it up. Sneezing follows, clearing out the mucus, and the adenoids will dry up.

An excellent composition powder is made as follows: All in powder form: bayberry bark 4 oz., African ginger 2 oz., hemlock spruce 1 oz., cloves 1 Dr., capsicum 1 Dr. Mix and pass through a fine sieve at least twice. The dose is 1 t. in 1 C. boiling water, sweetened. Cover and allow to stand a few minutes. Drink the clear liquid only.

This will raise the heat of the body, equalizing the circulation, and remove congestions, ease cramps and pains in the stomach and bowels, and is useful as a remedy in colds, beginning of fevers, flu, hoarseness, colic, clear canker of the stomach and bowels, and in acute fevers.

If this composition was kept in every home and used as the occasion arose, there would be less sickness. Take it freely. It is thoroughly safe and effective.

Where the circulation is weak and obstructed, when older people need a stimulating drink, and where the lumbar region is painful, an addition of 1 or 2 oz. of powdered white poplar bark will be helpful. It will also help the urinary tract.

As a drink for a gentle stimulation and to warm up the body, take ½ t. powder in 1 Cup boiling water, sweetened.

It is claimed that bayberry will prevent scrofula and tuberculosis.

The Thompson Compound is now prepared as a reliable fluid extract and also as an essence which can be quickly converted to an infusion by adding hot water; the powder may also be taken in capsule form, drinking hot water after. This will get rid of the disagreeable taste.

In all infusions, be sure to leave the powder and drink the liquid only.

BETH ROOT (Trillium Pendulum)

Beth root is a common plant growing in the Central and Western States.

It is also known as "birth root," a name given to it by the American Indians, who use it as an aid to parturition.

It influences the mucous membrane generally, especially that of the generative system. It is prompt and persistent but not drying. It will lessen excessive discharges, hence it is useful in excessive menstruation, leucorrhea, weak vagina, prolapsus uteri, and to prevent miscarriage. It is equally useful in hemorrhages, whether from the lungs, stomach, bowels, kidneys, bladder, uterine organs, or respiratory organs. A simple infusion will be of service in these conditions.

A good compound for prolapsus uteri and leucorrhea is equal parts of beth root and cranesbill, prepared either as an infusion or decoction. Take wine-glassful doses 4 to 5 times daily.

In languid cases, it will promote parturition, if taken previous to parturition. It will also anticipate hemorrhage.

Acute and chronic diarrhea and dysentery will be especially helped if the root is boiled in milk.

Beth root can be freely used to advantage in pulmonary

consumption, coughs, and in bronchial troubles. In coughs, 10 to 20 gr. of the powdered root may be taken in a little water 3 times daily.

A good antiseptic poultice may be made using 2 oz. each powdered beth root and powdered red elm, with ¼ oz. of powdered lobelia seed.

Boiling the LEAVES in lard will produce a good ointment useful for insect bites, etc.

The infusion is made with 1 t. powdered root to 1 C. boiling water. Drink freely, hot or cold.

BITTER ROOT (*Apocynum Androsemifolium*)

Bitter root is a native of the U.S. and flourishes in all parts of it. The ROOT is the part employed. Its taste is unpleasant and intensely bitter. It yields its medicinal properties to alcohol, but especially to water. Age impairs its medicinal quality.

Bitter root was a popular remedy among the Indians for syphilis. It is used today when the hepatic organs are sluggish.

Its influence is slow but persistent and extends through the gall ducts, gall cyst, liver tubuli and also the muscular and mucous membranes of the bowels and kidneys.

It is quite stimulating to the gall ducts, influencing the excretion of bile, and especially valuable when the stools are clay-colored, indicating a lack of bile. In jaundice, take 3 to 5 drops of the fluid extract every 2 or 3 hrs. and, if caused by occlusion, add American mandrake. If the pulse is below par, add a little capsicum. If using large doses for gall stones, add some ginger or aniseed.

Because it influences a discharge of bile and the bowels in the way it does, a soft stool will result in about 6 to 8 hrs. This is quite in order where torpid conditions are found, but is not good in irritated and sensitive conditions.

A good liver compound is made as follows: All in powder, white poplar bark and golden seal 2 oz. each, bitter root 1½ oz., culvers root and ginger ½ oz. each, capsicum ¼ oz. Mix and fill into #2 capsules and take 2 after each meal.

Bitter root is recommended in dropsy and hepatic troubles. In dropsy, combine bitter root with couch grass, gravel root, or juniper, taking 5 to 8 drops of the fluid extract every 2 to 4 hours.

As a cardiac stimulant in cardiac dropsy, take doses of 5 to 15 gr.

As a vermifuge, bitter root is most valuable; either alone or with golden seal. If taking the fluid extract, disguise the taste with a little compound syrup of rhubarb.

Used against the biting of a mad dog *(Hydrophobia)*, this plant was given the name of Dogbane.

All parts of the plant contain a milky juice, therefore it was also given the name "milkweed."

The down that is found in the cods of the plant was once used to make a soft stuffing for cushions and pillows.

BONESET *(Eupatorium Perfoliatum)*—Feverwort

According to the *Encyclopedia of Gardening*, the name "eupatorium" commemorates Mithridates Eupator, King of Pontus, who is credited with discovering that one of this species could be used as an antidote for poison.

It is also claimed that this plant caused a rapid union of broken bones, and because of this, it was given the name of boneset. However, it is more likely it was named for its wonderful efficacy in curing what was, at one time, called "breakbone fever," which is today called influenza. The Indians called it "Joe-Pie," after an Indian of that name who became famous in curing fevers with this plant. It is also a favorite remedy for the PREVENTION of fever.

Indigenous to the U.S., boneset grows in almost all parts of it.

All parts of the plant are active medicinally, and the entire HERB is official. It is considered a very reliable medicinal agent. It has a faint odor and a strongly bitter, somewhat peculiar taste. The bitterness, and probably the medicinal virtues of the plant, reside in an extractive matter which is readily taken up by water and alcohol.

This herb, best when it first blooms, is slow in its action but almost certain to relieve the liver. In large doses it is gently cathartic and gently tonic to the bowels throughout. It is invaluable in colds, fevers, and asthma.

It is said that the Indians successfully employed boneset in the cure of intermittents. It will certainly arrest intermittents when given freely in a warm decoction immediately before the expected recurrence of the paroxysms; but it is operated, in this instance, by its emetic rather than its tonic power.

It is claimed that the persistent use of this herb has PREVENTED many a case of typhoid and remitting fevers, and if not entirely prevented, it has made them much lighter than they would otherwise have been.

Use warm infusion in biliousness, bilious remitting fevers, yellow, and typhoid fever; the effect upon the liver and the bowels will be well marked. Taken in strong doses so as to produce vomiting or copious perspiration in the commencement of catarrh, it will frequently arrest that complaint.

For enteric (typhoid) fever, combine the following: boneset, twin leaf, prickly ash, false unicorn 1 oz. each. Simmer in 3 pints water 20 min. Strain and take 2 to 4 T. every hour or two as needed.

If a torpid liver causes the tongue to be foul, take a hot infusion of the above.

For chronic ague, boneset cannot be excelled.

In the epidemic of 1891, the following was used on 700 cases of la grippe, influenza, or epidemic catarrh (or whatever the popular name was at that time): boneset and false boneset 1½ oz. each, vervain, culvers root and agrimony 1 oz. each. He used the elixirs and gave 1 T. every 2 or 3 hours, as required. These herbs can be made into an infusion of 1 oz. to 1 pint boiling water. Take 2 to 4 T. every 2 or 3 hours. This is considered a very reliable formula.

Boneset has much value in many liver complaints and in bilious conditions, as it promotes secretion of bile by the liver and also stimulates the excretion of bile by the gall cysts.

If the bowels are too free as the result of torpor of the liver, use boneset. Also in acute and chronic jaundice. When the liver and the bowels both need help in constipation, use boneset and butternut in equal parts. This can be used either in powder form filled into capsules or made into an infusion. Not only will the liver be toned, but the butternut will influence the lower bowels, and good alvine action will result.

The following is a pleasant and extremely reliable compound for constipation, which can be continued as long as necessary: FX boneset and FX butternut 1 oz. each, and syrup ginger 4 oz. Take in t. doses, 3 or 4 times daily.

It is valuable in the treatment of rheumatism and inflammatory rheumatism, especially of the gouty and bilious classes.

In dyspeptic troubles, especially with constipation and general debility, a cold decoction will strengthen and tone the viscera.

For cerebro-spinal meningitis, the following is recommended: All elixirs—boneset 3 oz., vervain ½ oz., lady's slipper, black cohosh and culvers root, 1 oz. each and prickly ash ½ oz. Take 1 dessert-spoonful every 2 hrs. Also take a hot sponge bath, and if the bowels are constipated, use an enema.

Boneset is almost a specific in night sweats, especially in phthisis. Make a strong decoction of the herb in water, boil down to a solid extract, and make into pills. Take 1 pill every 1 to 3 hrs. This is also good in indigestion.

For its tonic effect, boneset is best taken in substance or cold infusion. Dose of the infusion is a fluid oz. frequently repeated. When a diaphoretic operation is required, the infusion should be taken warm and the patient remain covered in bed. As an emetic and cathartic, a strong decoction is prepared by boiling an oz. with 3 half pints of water down to 1 pt. May be taken in doses of 1 or 2 C. or more.

BURDOCK (*Arctium Lappa*)

This plant is a native of Europe. It grows wild in the northern parts of the U.S. and is also cultivated. The botanical name is from a Celtic word meaning "hand," because it catches at everything with which is comes in contact.

Only 1 yr. old roots should be used. The leaves and the stems are bitter, while the ROOTS and the SEEDS are somewhat sweet to the taste.

Burdock is considered one of the finest blood purifiers in the herbal system without irritating or nauseating properties. It will slowly influence the skin, soothe the kidneys, and relieve the lymphatics. It is recommended in gouty, scorbutic, venereal, rheumatic, scrofulous, leprous, and nephritic affection.

The SEEDS serve to better advantage than the ROOTS in dropsy, as they are more prompt in manifesting their influence. They will increase the flow of urine and are of service in irritation and inflammation of the bladder, scalding urine, and where a mucous discharge is found in the kidneys and urine. The seeds should be ground or bruised in order to obtain their properties quickly. In hot infusion, they influence the sebaceous glands and are of superior importance in scarlatina, typhoid fever, and other eruptive diseases.

The bruised seeds, 1 oz. simmered in 1½ pts. water down to 1 pt., strained and taken cold in doses of ⅓ to ½ teacupful 3 times daily, are said to be an unfailing remedy in almost all kidney troubles.

In skin troubles, such as rashes, pimples, boils, scurvy, and eczema, the root will give excellent results. It is said that burdock alone has cured eczema. It can be used internally or externally. In these troubles, yellow dock is considered a good addition, bathing the parts affected with a warm decoction frequently and drinking it warm at the same time, 4 to 6 wineglasses daily.

A fine remedy for the itching skin is made as follows: Simmer slowly for 2 hrs., 1# each fresh grated burdock root and leaf lard, 4 oz. suet and 1 oz. bee's wax. Strain and apply to the affected parts night and morning, at the same time drinking freely of the decoction of the root made of 1 oz. to 1 pint water.

Where there is also derangement of the nervous system, the seeds will have a soothing influence on the nerves.

Burdock root can be substituted for Sarsaparilla or sanicle.

Both root and seed may be taken as a decoction, considered the best form of administration, made of 1 oz. to 1½ pts. water boiled down to 1 pt. and taken in doses of 1 wine-glassful 3 or 4 times daily.

Dr. Robinson writes: Remember that a kind Providence has made some of the most useful plants the most common.

BUTTERNUT (Juglans Cinerea)
An indigenous forest tree, butternut grows throughout most of the U.S. The hardwood is used for furniture and interior trim. The bark is used for dying wool a dark-brown color. The fruit, when half grown, is made into pickles, and when ripe, it is used as a food.

The INNER BARK is the medical portion and that of the ROOT is considered the best. It has a feeble odor and a peculiarly bitter, somewhat acrid taste. Its medicinal virtues are extracted by boiling water, except its astringency, which it yields to alcohol.

Butternut is a mild cathartic, operating without pain or irritation and resembling rhubarb in evacuating without debilitating the alimentary canal. It was highly esteemed and much employed as a laxative by the Army during the Revolutionary War.

The alcoholic extract sold by the druggist may be used in diarrhea and dysentery.

The liquid extract is very valuable in chronic constipation. It will tone the entire alvine membrane, being particularly tonic to the lower bowels, influencing peristalsis.

It is moderately slow, operating in 4 to 8 hours, but very reliable. It relieves the portal circulation, especially where the liver is engorged. It will bring about the ejection of bile and the cleansing of the hepatic and alvine accumulations, but it will not bring about watery evacuations.

It is considered of excellent service in habitual constipation and other bowel affections, particularly dysentery, in which it has acquired considerable reputation.

A simple syrup of butternut can be made as follows: Fl X butternut ½ oz., 4 oz. sugar, and 10 oz. boiling water. Mix and bottle. Dose is 1 T. twice daily, children in proportion.

This syrup is excellent for hemorrhoids and rectal hemorrhage. FE stone root may be added.

For tapeworm, it is considered a reliable remedy, especially for children.

The oil may be applied to irritated sores.

Butternut is usually taken in the form of decoction or extract. The extract is official, and is always preferred. The dose is from 20 to 30 gr. as a purge, from 5 to 10 gr. as a laxative.

The solid extract is used either in pills or syrup, 4 or 5 pills taken at night.

CASCARA SAGRADA (*Rhamnus Purshiana*)

A tree growing on the shores of the Pacific. An old Indian remedy, it was called by them "sacred bark." It should be one year old before using. The BARK is the official portion. The taste is persistently bitter.

Its range of influence includes the stomach, liver, gall ducts, and bowels, specifically the lower bowels. In habitual and chronic constipation where the lower bowel is at fault, cascara will influence peristaltic action, also in torpor of the stomach and liver and in chronic dyspepsia, and is especially helpful where hemorrhoids or piles are found.

Where a gentle laxative is needed, take small doses of fluid extract from 20–25 drops 3 times daily.

Where prompt action is desired on the lower bowel, take fluid extract ½ to ¾ Dr. and then smaller doses 3 times daily until the desired result is obtained.

Many laxatives and cathartics lose their effects if taken frequently. This is not so with cascara.

The fluid extract is used to a great extent and represents the bark fully.

CAYENNE *(Capsicum Annum)*

The African bird pepper *(Capsicum Baccatum)*, from the W. Indies and So. America, is considered the purest and best stimulant known. CAPSICUM ANNUM is extensively cultivated in this country, and although a large quantity is imported from the West Indies, it is considered official in the U.S.

When perfectly ripe and dry, the fruit is ground into powder and brought into market under the name of red or cayenne pepper. The odor is peculiar and somewhat aromatic, stronger in the fresh than the dried fruit. The taste is bitter and produces a fiery sensation in the mouth, which continues for a long time.

It is much employed as a condiment by the natives of tropical climates, who live chiefly on vegetables, to correct the flatulent tendency of certain vegetables and to bring them within the digestive powers of the stomach. In the East Indies, it has been used from time immemorial and has also been known to the Romans.

In this country, it is used as a condiment in many dishes such as salads, dressings, sauces, fish, cheese, eggs, and curries. It is very nutritious and is pure vitamin C, and contains calcium, phosphorus, iron, and also vitamins A, B_1, and G.

As a medicine, it is useful in all cases requiring a stimulant.

Cayenne pepper is a powerful stimulant and produces, when swallowed, a sense of heat in the stomach and a general warmth over the whole body, without any narcotic effect.

The fruit is the most positive and persistent heart stimulant known and is exceedingly prompt in its effect. By equalizing the circulation, it influences the whole body; the heart first, next the arteries, the capillaries, and then the nerves.

It is useful in failing and sluggish circulation, sinking spells, dysentery, bilious colic, cholera and cholera infantum, paralysis, pleurisy, aphonia, gastric catarrh, gangrene, typhoid fever, palsy, yellow fever, shock from injury, and where there are cold and clammy sweats.

The Negroes of the West Indies soak the pods in water, add sugar and the juice of sour oranges, and drink freely in fevers.

In cases of apoplexy, it is known to give good results when the feet are placed into a hot bath with mustard and ½ t. cayenne added. The pressure is removed from the brain, and the circulation equalized.

In cramps, pain in the stomach and bowels, and in constipation, it will create heat and cause peristaltic action. Use small doses of the warm infusion of ½ to 1 t. to 1 C. boiling water.

Cayenne is very useful in inflammations.

In typhoid fever, add a little golden seal and an hepatic to sustain the portal circulation and to increase the value of the hepatic.

In colds, relaxed throat, cold conditions of the stomach, enfeebled and languid stomach, dyspepsia, and atonic gout, particularly with flatulence occurring in persons of intemperate habits, spasms, palpitation, particularly in the acute stages, take a warm infusion in small repeated doses about 2 t. every ½ hour or more frequently, if required.

For cold feet, sprinkle a LITTLE capsicum inside your shoes or socks. When exposed to cold and damp for any length of time, take pills or capsules of pure cayenne.

In hemorrhage from the lungs, use a vapor bath and an infusion of cayenne; pressure will be taken from the ruptured blood vessels.

In quinsy and diphtheria, wet a cloth with the infusion or tincture of cayenne, place around the neck, and cover with flannel or wool. Drink the infusion at the same time and gargle, or spray, the inside of the throat with an atomizer.

Its most important application is in the treatment of malignant sore throat and scarlet fever, in which it is used both internally and as a gargle. No other remedy can claim equal credit in these conditions.

The following is a formula originated in the West Indies where it is used to great advantage in malignant scarlatina: Infuse 2 T. powdered cayenne with 1 t. common salt for 1 hr. in 1 pt. boiling liquid composed of equal parts of water and vinegar; strain; take 1 T. every ½ hr. This is also used as a gargle. In milder cases with inflamed or ulcerated throat, take a more diluted dose.

For sprains, bruises, rheumatism, and neuralgia, a liniment is more effective if cayenne is added, or cayenne may be applied externally as a plaster.

The powder or tincture brought into contact with a relaxed uvula is often very beneficial.

Cayenne reduces dilated blood vessels in those addicted to alcohol.

In cases of severe congestions, cayenne may be added to the bath water.

Internally capsicum may be taken in infusions, in syrups, in fluid extract, in water, or the oil may be mixed in sugar. Take small doses frequently and wait for the cumulative results.

The dose of the powder is from 5 to 10 grains in pill form. An infusion can be prepared by adding 2 dr. to ½ pt. boiling water; the dose is about ½ fl. oz.

Increase the dose of cayenne as vitality decreases.

If the application of capsicum gives much burning sensation, use some lard or other oil over the surface.

WILD CARROT *(Daucus carota)*

The umbel of this plant is concave like a bird's nest, and from this came the name of "bird's nest." It is also known as Queen Anne's lace.

The wild carrot is exceedingly common in the U.S. It also grows wild in Europe, and is believed by some botanists to have been introduced into the U.S. The well-known garden carrot is the same plant, although somewhat altered by cultivation. The official portions are the SEEDS of the wild and the ROOTS of the cultivated variety.

Carrot seeds have an aromatic odor and a warm, pungent, and bitterish taste. By distillation, they yield a pale yellow volatile oil, upon which their virtues chiefly depend. Boiling water extracts their active properties.

The seeds are moderately excitant and diuretic, and are used considerably, both in domestic practice and by physicians, in chronic nephritic affections and in dropsy. As they possess some of the cordial properties of the aromatics, they are especially adapted to cases in which the stomach is enfeebled. From 30 gr. to a drachm. of the bruised seeds may be taken as a dose; or a pint of the infusion made of ½ oz. or 1 oz. of the seeds, taken during the day. The whole umbel is often used instead of the seeds alone.

The root of the wild carrot is whitish, hard, resembling leather, branched, has a strong smell and an acrid disagreeable taste; that of the cultivated variety is reddish, fleshy, thick, conical, rarely branched, of a pleasant odor and, a sweet, mucilaginous, yet peculiar taste, dependent on the presence of saccharine and gummy matters that have been detected in considerable quantity to render the root nutritious.

The wild root possesses the same medicinal properties as the seeds and has much reputation as an external application to gangrenous, and sloughing ulcers. Boiled and mashed, the root is applied in the form of a plaster.

The entire wild plant is used and is highly valued as a diuretic in the treatment of dropsy, affections of the bladder, gravel, stricture, retention of urine, or any obstruction of the urinary passages or bladder.

It has a favorable influence upon the stomach, removing coldness and flatulence. It may be given either in infusion or decoction.

The cultivated carrot root of our gardens is sweeter and is well-known as a food; it has, however, other uses as well. It has been found a most useful article as a stimulating application for sores, ulcers, abscesses, carbuncles, and scrofulous sores. It should be grated and applied raw. It has a cleansing effect and stimulates the part to sound granulation after which other healing agents will make a more favorable impression.

Do not continue the wild or cultivated carrot after full vital action in the part has come about; use other healing methods then.

The following is recommended in dropsy: wild carrot and hair cap moss 1½ oz. each, crushed watermelon seeds 1 oz. Simmer in 3 pts. water for 20 min. Strain and take 2 T. every 2 hours and use the vapor bath 2 or 3 times a week.

The infusion of 1 oz. to 1 pt. boiling water is taken in wineglassful doses.

CATNIP *(Nepeta cataria)*

Catnip is a common garden plant. Its odor and taste is mintlike and strongly aromatic. It gets its name from the fact that cats like to eat it and roll themselves in it.

It is claimed our early settlers taught the American Indians how to make catnip tea, and that it has remained a favorite with them. They claimed it brought on sound and restful sleep.

Though considered for many years a good remedy for children, its usefulness is by no means limited to the troubles of children. It is, however, a very important remedy in children's colic, restlessness, nervous irritability, and fevers.

An injection of the infusion of the HERB will speedily overcome convulsions in children, also in restlessness and colic. Just sweeten an infusion and inject 1 C. at body temperature. The colic will be eased, and a restless child will be quieted.

This injection is also very beneficial in hysteria and nervous headache.

In invagination of the bowels, use a strong infusion as an injection. Use constantly, possibly 2 or 3 gallons, until relieved. It is claimed there is nothing better.

A hot infusion, through its influence upon the circulation, will produce perspiration. The addition of a little ginger will intensify the effect. It will be useful in colds, soothe the nervous system, relieve irritation, and increase the menstrual and urine flow.

In feverish colds, taken hot upon retiring, it will induce peaceful sleep.

For fevers with depressed or low vitality, the following is considered an excellent compound: catnip, pleurisy root and lobelia herb 1 oz. each, composition powder ½ oz., all in fine powder. Mix well together. Place 1 t. in 1 C. boiling water, sweeten, cover, and allow to stand a few minutes. Take ¼ C. warm every 1½ hr. for an adult and children in proportion.

This herb is considered of some use against barrenness.

Legend tells us that a tea made from the leaves of catnip gives courage to the timid and makes the weak strong.

AMERICAN CENTAURY *(Sabbatia angularis)*

This plant grows in moist meadows in most of the U.S. It is considered preferable to the European centaury *(Erytherea Centaurium)* which it closely resembles.

The whole HERB is used and should be collected when in flower. All parts of it have a strongly bitter taste without astringency or peculiar flavor. Both alcohol and water extract its bitterness and its medicinal virtues.

American centaury has the tonic properties of the simple bitters. It has long been popularly employed as a preventive and protective remedy in our autumnal intermittent and remittent fevers. The state of fever to which it is particularly applicable is that which exists in the intervals between the paroxysms, when the remissions are such as to call for the use of tonics, but not sufficiently decided to justify a resort to Peruvian bark.

It is useful during a slow convalescence by promoting appetite and invigorating the digestive function, and may be used in dyspepsia and general debility.

The most convenient form of use is that of infusion made of 1 pt. boiling water on 1 oz. HERB and allowed to cool. May be taken in doses of 2 fl. oz., repeated every hour, or two during the remission of fevers and less frequently in chronic affections. The dose of the powder is from 30 gr. to 1 Dr. The decoction, extract, and the tincture are also efficient preparations.

This HERB is a positive, diffusive stimulating tonic to the heart, stomach, liver, generative organs, and the nervous system.

In hot infusion, it promotes menstruation and influences a good outward circulation.

ROMAN CHAMOMILE *(Anthemis nobilis)*

A native of Europe, Roman chamomile grows wild in some parts of this country. It is largely cultivated for medicinal purposes.

The whole HERB is used. However, the double flowers have been used chiefly in medicine, much of it being imported from Germany and England. Although the double flowers are preferred, the yellow flower discs contain the valuable medicinal properties and not being fully developed in the double flowers, the single are the most powerful. The radial florets contain the aromatic flavor: the whitest (when dried) are preferred. The FLOWERS only are official.

The Roman chamomile is considered the true chamomile, although the German chamomile (*Matricaria Chamomilia*), belonging to the same family, is closely allied in medicinal properties.

The whole HERB has a peculiar odor and a bitter aromatic taste. The flowers impart their odor and taste to both water and alcohol. They are known to contain an essential oil, probably one of their active ingredients. It may be obtained by distilling the flowers with water.

Chamomile is a mild tonic and in small doses strengthens the stomach. In cold infusion, it is advantageously used in enfeebled digestion and indigestion. It is especially applicable to cases of general debility with languid appetite, which often attends convalescence from idiopathic fevers. For digestive troubles, infuse 5 or 6 of the flowers in ½ C. boiling water, allow to stand a few minutes, then drink the whole.

Chamomile has acquired a reputation as a febrifuge, especially in remittants when the subsidence of action between the paroxysms is so considerable as to demand the use of tonics but not sufficiently complete to resort to Peruvian Bark.

Chamomile, in substance, has, in some instances, proved effectual in the treatment of intermittents.

The tepid infusion is often given to promote emetic medicines or to assist the stomach in relieving itself when oppressed by its contents. Large and frequent doses will cause an emesis, but this will be an advantage rather than a detriment.

The flowers are sometimes applied as fomentations in irritation or inflammation of the abdominal viscera and as gentle incitants in flabby, ill-conditioned ulcers.

The infusion is usually preferred. The decoction and extract cannot exert the full influence of the medicine, as the essential oil, upon which its virtues partly depend, is drawn off at the boiling temperature.

The hot infusion will produce a good flow of blood to the surface. It acts promptly upon the circulation, stomach, nerves,

28

mucous membrane, and uterus. It is useful in colds, bilious fevers, puerperal fever, and bilious headache.

The cold infusion will be useful in amenorrhoea and dysemenorrhoea when the menstrual flow is slow and painful causing nervous irritation, it acting upon the uterus in relieving congestion and stimulating the flow. In colds, the warm or hot infusion with the addition of a little ginger will be found effective. In coughs, where a soothing expectorant is needed, add spikenard.

A poultice of the FLOWERS is excellent in the reduction of swellings where it is not desirable to bring them to a head.

The following has been widely used in the treatment of painful bruises, swellings, neuralgia and toothache: chamomile flowers 1 oz. and 3 poppy heads. Break the poppy heads and mix together. Pour on sufficient boiling water to make into a poultice and apply as hot as possible.

It was once thought if consumptives breathed in the odor of the chamomile, it would have a purifying effect on the lungs.

Hairdressers use the flowers to rinse the hair, to preserve the golden tints, and to add to its fragrance. Oil is used in hair lotions. To make the hair rinse, simmer the flowers for 1 hr. then strain and bottle for use.

As a tonic, the powdered flowers may be used in doses of ½ to 1 Dr., 3 times daily. The infusion of 1 oz. to 1 pint boiling water is taken in doses of 1 T. to 1 wine-glassful.

The flowers should NEVER be boiled as the volatile oil will escape in the steam.

WILD CHERRY (Prunus virginiana)

In 1833, Botanist Michaux claims he saw, on the banks of the Ohio, wild cherry trees from 80' to 100' high with trunks 12' to 15' in circumference and undivided to the height of 25' to 30'. However, the tree, as we know it, is usually of much smaller dimensions.

This tree grows throughout the U.S. It is highly valued by cabinet-makers for its wood, which is compact, fine-grained, susceptible of polish, and of a light red tint which deepens with age.

The fruit has a sweetish, astringent, bitter taste, and is much employed in some parts of the country to impart flavor to liquors.

The inner BARK is the part employed in medicine and is obtained indiscriminately from all parts of the tree, although that of the roots is most active. The young thin bark is the best. It is preferred recently dried, as it deteriorates by keeping.

In the fresh state, or when boiled in water, it emits an odor resembling that of peach leaves. Its taste is agreeably bitter and aromatic, with the peculiar flavor of the bitter almond.

It imparts its medicinal properties to water, either cold or hot, producing a clear reddish infusion closely resembling Madeira wine in appearance. Its peculiar flavor is injured by boiling in consequence of the volatilization of the principle upon which it depends.

This bark is among the most valuable of the botanic remedies and long an old home remedy for cough syrup.

It is a mild, soothing, astringent tonic to the mucous membrane, especially of the respiratory organs, the pelvic, and the alvine canal.

As a tonic and expectorant, it is considered of the highest value in catarrhal affections, nervous excitement in consumption, consumption, in acute, irritable, and nervous coughs, whooping cough, bronchitis, diseases of the chest and lungs, and in fact, in all diseases of the respiratory organs; it quiets nervous irritability and relieves arterial excitement.

When largely taken, it is said to diminish the action of the heart. If a good portion of the cold infusion is taken several times a day and continued for nearly 2 weeks, it should reduce the pulse from 75 to 50 strokes in the minute.

It is a favorite remedy and highly useful in the hectic fever of scrofula and consumption and as a tonic in the convalescence from fevers.

It has been used successfully in intermittent fever, but in this complaint is considered inferior to Peruvian Bark.

In the general debility which often succeeds inflammatory diseases, it has also been found advantageous and is well adapted to many cases of dyspepsia. It is equally valuable in gastritis and atonic conditions of the digestive organs.

A fine powder inhaled as snuff will benefit a moist catarrh and also the lungs.

The fresh bark is preferred. Ground and in fine powder put into a self-sealing jar, pour boiling hot syrup over it and seal.

Let stand a few days. This makes an excellent syrup of prunus.

Wild cherry bark may be used in powder or infusion. The dose of the powder is from 30 gr. to 1 Dr. The simple infusion is prepared with 1 t. inner bark to 1 C. boiling water. Drink cold 1 or 2 C. daily.

CHICKWEED *(Stellaria media)*

This plant, considered a curse by many gardeners because of its creeping and twining among other plants, is worth its weight in gold.

It is a good nutritious food which can be eaten raw as a salad or cooked the same as any other vegetable. The seeds provide food for the birds and poultry. Its taste is slightly saline, with no odor.

In all chest troubles, in inflammation of the lungs, bowels, or stomach, bronchitis, asthma, in the bleeding of the lungs or bowels, in peritonitis and in other internal inflammatory conditions, chickweed is highly recommended boiled, eaten, and the water drunk freely. It has an extremely soothing and healing influence.

It is of value in debilitated conditions, anemia, consumption, and rheumatism. It is claimed that consumptive people and children suffering from malnutrition will quickly gain strength if this herb is used as a food.

In blood poisoning, the decoction taken internally and a chickweed poultice applied locally, is said to be very effective.

Chickweed will give good results in external applications. In swollen testicles, tumors, all external inflamed surfaces, sores and skin diseases, eruptions and irritations, make a strong decoction and wash the parts affected with it twice a day, at least, and apply chickweed ointment. It is a valuable and reliable remedy. It can also be taken internally at the same time.

The fresh leaves have been used with good results as a poultice in indolent ulcers.

In erysipelas, no matter how bad the pain and swelling, boil a handful or 2 of chickweed and bathe the surface every ½ hr. and apply chickweed ointment. Within a few hours, the pain and the swelling should be relieved.

The ointment is said to alleviate the burning and itching around the genitals.

The ointment is made as follows: 1# fresh green chickweed, 1½# leaf lard or vegetable shortening, 2 oz. bee's wax. Cut the chickweed, add other ingredients. Cover and render in the oven 3 hrs., then strain. When cold, it is ready for use.

Chickweed may be used fresh or dried; in powder, decoction, infusion, poultice, fomentation, or in ointment.

CLIVERS (*Galium aperine*)

Clivers is a plant common all over the U.S. It has an unpleasant odor, which is lost when dried, and has an acidulous, astringent, and bitter taste. Cold or warm water extracts its virtues.

Clivers influences the kidneys and bladder, and thus is excellent in gravel, scalding urine, and irritation at the neck of the bladder. In the suppression of urine and obstruction of the urinary organs, it increases the urine, relieves the irritated bladder and urethra, and in the inflammatory stage of gonorrhea, it relieves the irritation and soothes the nervous system.

In acute gonorrhea, take from ½ to a whole fluid oz. of the fresh juice every 4 to 6 hours.

The expressed juice is useful applied to sore nipples and sores. It exercises great control over diseases of the skin. Tablespoon doses of the expressed juice can be taken 3 times a day.

A tea made from this herb is considered good for the dropsy, not only as a diuretic, but also for its aperient properties, as it acts mildly upon the bowels. It is equally useful in cases of scrofula, and long standing ulcers. Take 2 oz. of the expressed juice 3 times a day and apply a poultice of the green herb.

It is quite a solvent of stone in the bladder and has been used as a specific in scurvy.

In hot infusion, this plant may be used to good advantage in fevers.

It should, when possible, be taken in infusion. The infusion, hot or cold, of 1 oz. to 1 pt. boiling water is taken frequently in wine-glassful doses.

It is a very powerful diuretic and therefore should NOT be used where there is a tendency to diabetes.

A permanent red dye is obtained from the roots of clivers.

RED CLOVER (*Trifolium pratense*)

Red clover is the state flower of Vermont.

The FLOWERS should be gathered in perfect bloom, and if desired, dried and packed for use later. The taste and odor is agreeable.

Red clover is very useful in spasmodic, bronchial, and whooping coughs, usually by infusion.

The warm infusion is soothing to the nerves and is mildly laxative to the bowels. The hot infusion influences the circulation to a good capillary distribution.

A good compound alterative is made by combining red clover, burdock, yellow parilla each 1 oz., and ½ oz. mullein. Simmer in 2 quarts water down to 1 quart. Strain and take a wine-glassful 3 or 4 times daily.

Red clover has quite an old reputation as a wash for scaly skins and the solid extract is a highly recommended application for indolent ulcers. It promotes healthy granulation.

The infusion of 1 oz. to 1 pt. boiling water may be used freely.

BLACK COHOSH (Cimicifuga racemosa)

Black cohosh is a native of the U.S. growing in shady and rocky woods from Canada to Florida.

It is also called black snakeroot, squaw root, and bugbane. The name black snakeroot was probably derived from its supposed power of curing the bite of the rattlesnake. The name of squawroot was given to it because it was thought by some to have a particular affinity for the uterus. The name of bugbane was given to it because its name came from *cimex,* meaning a bug and *fugo,* meaning to drive away. It is said the leaves drive away bugs.

The ROOT is the part used. The color is externally dark brown, almost black, internally whitish; the odor is disagreeable but is almost entirely absent when dry; the taste is bitter and somewhat astringent, leaving a slight sense of acrimony. The root yields its virtues to boiling water only partially but wholely to alcohol.

Black cohosh is useful employed as a remedy in dropsy, hysteria, and various affections of the lungs, particularly those resembling consumption, hysterical, and puerperal convulsions and asthma.

Its influence on the nerves is very gradual, but at the same time it is a powerful remedy, soothing and relieving local pains, and is of use in general nervous excitement. In insomnia and headache, where the pain is felt at the back of the head and the base of the brain, the infusion in small doses will bring relief.

Black cohosh soothes the serous membrane, gives a fullness to the pulse, and is therefore of much importance in acute and chronic rheumatism.

While black cohosh is said to be a specific in the treatment of chorea of children and rheumatism, it is without doubt a most valuable remedy in pelvic disturbances. In uterine troubles, its influence is quite marked, and it relieves rheumatism of that organ. It soothes the uterus, and in retention of and painful menstruation and in parturition it is very efficient. When the menstrual flow is retarded by cold or exposure, the warm infusion is most dependable. An addition of blue cohosh, in equal parts, is helpful.

The following nerve tonic is useful for epilepsy and chorea: All Fl. Ex., black cohosh 4 oz., skullcap, and valerian of each 2 oz., simple syrup 4 oz. Dose 1 T. 4 times daily. All meats and heavy indigestible foods should be strictly avoided.

A syrup is made by adding enough sugar to a decoction of the fresh or dried roots to keep it. The syrup may be very well used as a base for alterative compounds, tonics, and antispasmodics, and gives favorable results. In eruptive diseases as in scrofula and smallpox, the syrup may be taken freely for a day or 2 when it will be found to be of great value. It will tend to purify the blood current so that the eruption will not be so virulent and the surface inflammation not so intense.

The syrup acts well on the secernents throughout the liver, kidneys, and lymphatics. It is a good remedy in syphilis.

It is also given in coughs and in whooping coughs. Small doses are useful in children's diarrhea.

In violent outburst of consumption, black cohosh will give relief by allaying the cough, reducing rapidity of the pulse, and inducing perspiration.

In apoplexy, try the following: Fl. X. black cohosh and Fl. X. wood betony 1 oz. each, tincture of cayenne 2 Dr. Take 1 t. every 10 min. until improvement is indicated and then every hour or 2. Meanwhile place the feet in hot water with mustard and cayenne. After removing the feet from the bath, place a hot water bottle wrapped in a flannel wrung out of vinegar to the feet. An injection of lobelia, skullcap and cayenne about ¼ t. ea. in ¾ pint warm water injected about the warmth of fresh milk will help. The object is to remove the pressure from the brain. This will equalize the circulation. If the injection does not evacuate the bowels, repeat until the patient perspires freely.

The decoction is usually preferred, 1 oz. of the bruised root may be boiled for a short time in 1 pint water. Dose 1 or 2 fl. oz. several times daily.

The fluid X may be used either in hot or cold preparation. This cannot, however, be used in large quantities, but the syrup can be taken as often as required.

BLUE COHOSH (*Caulophyllum Thalictroides*)

Blue cohosh grows in rich moist ground in most of the U.S. The taste is sweetish, then bitter and acrid. It is nearly inodorous.

The American Indians called it "papoose root." The squaws used blue cohosh ROOT to expedite parturition and to induce menstruation.

Its chief influence is upon the generative system, also soothing and toning the nervous system.

In leucorrhea and amenorrhea, it will do good work. In dysmenorrhea, the antispasmodic properties will be used to excellent advantage. In puerperal convulsions, it will assist the flow which is usually suspended at that time. In the irritation of the nerves that frequently occurs during parturition and for false pains, the restlessness during pregnancy, and for after-pains, blue cohosh is superior.

In vaginitis, blue cohosh has a useful place if taken internally and used as an injection to the vagina. It is excellent in uterine irritation.

In urethritis, whether of the male or of the female, it prevents too frequent urination and soothes the irritation.

It can be used safely in cases where it is desirable to relax the muscle fibre. It is valuable in fits, cramps, colic, and spasms.

In hysteria, it will soothe the nervous irritation and an addition of skullcap will furnish greater tone.

Its antispasmodic powers will be of value in spasmodic asthma and whooping and catarrhal coughs. Blue cohosh may be added to spikenard and wild cherry in cough syrups. Adding wild ginger is said to be a specific in whooping cough.

In bronchial catarrh, the following is a good combination: blue cohosh and comfrey root 1 oz. each, pleurisy root ½ oz., lobelia 2 dr., ginger ¼ oz. Infuse in 1 qt. boiling water. Cover and keep warm 20 min. Strain and take 1 to 2 T. 3 or 4 times daily.

For rheumatism and neuralgia, blue cohosh is used extensively.

For Chorea, after-pains and nervousness during parturition use: 3 parts wild yam, 2 parts blue cohosh, 1 part skullcap.

For rigidity of the os uteri, add a little lobelia to the above.

A simple infusion is made of 1 t. root to 1 C. boiling water. Drink cold during the day.

COLTSFOOT *(Tussilago Farfara)*

This plant grows wild upon the banks of streams, rivers, and wet places in the Middle and Northern United States.

The LEAVES are most frequently employed, and they should be gathered after their full expansion. The FLOWERS have an agreeable odor which they retain if carefully dried. The dried ROOT and leaves are inodorous. When dried, all parts have a rough, bitter, mucilaginous, slightly astringent taste. Boiling water or diluted alcohol extracts all their medicinal virtues.

Coltsfoot is also called coughwort, and is considered a very valuable HERB of use particularly in chronic coughs, colds, consumption, hoarseness, asthma, bronchitis, and whooping cough. It can be safely and effectively employed in all manner of lung troubles. It increases expectoration, tones the bronchi, and is valuable in debilitated pulmonary troubles. Coltsfoot is very soothing to the mucous membrane.

An infusion of coltsfoot, marshmallow, ground ivy and black horehound in equal parts will prove a reliable cough remedy.

A simple preparation for coughs and colds is made as follows: Boil 2 oz. leaves in 1½ pts. water 15 min. Strain and sweeten with 2 oz. honey. Take a wine-glassful 4 to 6 times daily. Children in proportion.

Poultices are made of the fresh leaves or the expressed juice may be applied externally, especially on scrofulous sores.

The leaves were smoked by the ancients in pulmonary complaints, and we are informed that even at the present time coltsfoot is substituted for tobacco in Europe.

An herbal tobacco is made by blending 2 parts coltsfoot leaves with 1 part each eyebright, rosemary, thyme, and lavender.

This can be used very effectively as a smoking tobacco in asthma.

Coltsfoot may be used either in infusion, decoction, powder, pills, or fluid extract. The usual form is that of a decoction; 1 oz. of the leaves or plant in 2 pts. water boiled down to 1 pt. of which 1 teacupful sweetened may be taken several times daily.

For a simple infusion, steep 1 t. leaves into 1 C. boiling water for ½ hr. Take 1 C. 3 times daily.

AMERICAN COLUMBO (*Frasera Carolinesis*)

Only one of its genus has been discovered. An indigenous plant, American columbo flourishes in the Southern and Western portion of the U.S. Because the stem and flowers are produced only in the 3rd year, the ROOT should be collected in the autumn of the second or the spring of the 3rd year. Before being dried, it should be cut into transverse slices.

The taste is somewhat bitter. Water and diluted alcohol extract their virtues.

American columbo is a mild, stimulating, slightly astringent tonic. It is sometimes used as a substitute for the foreign columbo. It has been thought to resemble it in medicinal properties as well as in appearance hence has received the popular name of American columbo.

The fresh root is said to operate as an emetic and cathartic, and is sometimes taken for this purpose.

Its chief influence is expended upon the alvine mucous membrane as a tonic, and it is therefore useful in cases of weak digestion and diarrhea, especially in children. It promotes appetite and aids digestion.

In gastric ulceration and gastric catarrh, American columbo is one of the most valuable and most reliable.

Combined with uterine remedies or vaginal tonics, it will expend its influence on these organs and is useful in prolapsis uteri, uterine and vaginal weakness, and ulceration.

An infusion forms an excellent vaginal wash for a weak vagina, prolapsus uteri, and leucorrhea. Also for aphthous sore mouth.

A good tonic for possible miscarriage can be made as follows: American columbo 3 oz., true unicorn root 2 oz., 1 oz. each of golden seal root, squaw vine (mitchella) and orange peel. Simmer in 3 qts. water for ½ hr. Strain and take 1 wine-glassful 3 or 4 times daily. This can also be used for foul leucorrhea.

American columbo is an excellent tonic in typhoid fever, and if troubled with diarrhea, it will give good results.

It may be taken in powder or infusion. The dose of the powder is from 30 grains to a drachm. The dose of the infusion, made in the proportion of 1 oz. of the bruised root to 1 pt. of boiling water, is 1 or 2 fl. oz., to be repeated several times a day. The fluid extract may be used.

COMFREY (Symphytum Officinalis)

Comfrey, a native of Europe, is now naturalized in the U.S. Its taste is sweet, mucilaginous, and faintly astringent with no odor. The ROOT contains a large amount of mucilage which is readily extracted by water.

It would be difficult to name a more useful herb. Because of its great healing power, it was given the name of "knit-bone."

It is a soothing demulcent and tonic to the mucous membrane, especially of the respiratory organs. It allays irritation, increases expectoration, and tones the bronchi.

It is a fairly safe rule to figure always to use comfrey root in coughs, colds, asthma, especially with excessive expectoration, tuberculosis, especially of the lung, ulcerated and inflamed lung conditions, hemorrhage, coughing up or spitting of blood, nasal congestion and catarrh, soreness of the stomach and bowels, and ulcerated kidneys.

Owing to its soothing effect, it is useful in diarrhea and dysentery.

When the urine is bloody and when gravel is suspected, use comfrey.

The fresh plant, leaves or root, bruised, is a good fomentation to bruises, sprains, irritated sores, obstinate ulcers, and inflammatory boils, especially in the supperation stage, swelling and fractures. It will reduce the swelling and ease the pain.

An excellent nervine cough syrup is made of 1 oz. each of the following: comfrey root, turkey rhubarb, elecampane rt., spikenard, skunk cabbage, and white horehound. Boil in 5 pts. water for 30 min., strain, then boil down the liquid to 1½ pts. Then, while hot, add 2# sugar. Cool. If it is desired to preserve it for any length of time, 1 oz. of alcohol should be added. The dose is 1 dessert-spoonful 3 or 4 times daily.

A very good lung tonic is made of ½ oz. each of the following: comfrey root, horehound, elecampane rt., ground ivy, ginger rt. and ½ t. cayenne. Simmer in 3 pts. of water 20 min., then add 2 t. powdered nutmeg. Cover and simmer 4 min. longer. Strain and add to the hot liquid 1½# sugar. Bottle when cold. Dose 1 or 2 T. every 2 hrs.

A decoction of the root is made by boiling ½ or 1 oz. crushed comfrey in 1 qt. water or milk. Dose is 1 wine-glassful. The leaves are usually made into an infusion.

CORN SILK (*Zea Mays*)

Indian corn is known to every American.

The fine, silky, yellowish threads, or CORN SILK, are the stigmas from the female flowers of maize. They must be gathered immediately after its pollen has been shed and before they become dry. They must be carefully dried and kept in a closed container to prevent evaporation of the oil upon which much of its medicinal virtues depend. The taste is sweet with no odor.

Corn silk is a soothing demulcent and tonic diuretic, and is considered a valuable remedy in many urinary and bladder conditions. It increases the flow of urine and is of special service in purulent decomposition of urine in the bladder. It will cleanse the cystic membrane in cystic catarrh and will manifest antiseptic powers in morbid deposits. It has a reputation for cleansing the circulation of urea and is valuable in the treatment of renal and cystic inflammation.

In cystitis: the following should give relief within a few hours: FE corn silk 1½ oz., FE uva ursi ½ oz., wintergreen 60 gr. Mix and take 1 t. every 1, 2 or 3 hrs. as needed.

Corn silk will soothe the kidneys and bladder and relieve the urine of that strong odor of ammonia which is sometimes present.

Not being possible to use within a few hours after being gathered, it is more convenient to use the fluid extract as placed upon the market. The infusion of 1 pt. boiling water is a most active preparation and should be taken freely.

CRAMP BARK (*Viburnum Opulus*)

Although this plant is also known as high cranberry, it is in no sense a species of the edible cranberry.

It is indigenous to the Northern part of the U.S. The BARK

is the official part. It has no odor. The taste is somewhat bitter and slightly astringent. It yields its properties to water or diluted alcohol.

It is a splendid antispasmodic and, as the name cramp bark implies, it is good in cramps. It will speedily relieve the pains of cramps in limbs in pregnancy and where any nervous troubles are in evidence due to the pregnant state, it is useful. It will prevent miscarriage. For even better results add wild yam, blue cohosh, squaw vine, or skullcap.

In painful menstruation and when rheumatic pains are felt in the uterine region, cramp bark is very useful. It is the best relaxant to the ovaries and uterus.

Also can be used with much success in fits, fainting, neuralgia, lockjaw, flatulent-stomach, convulsions, and spasms of all kinds.

May be taken either in decoction or infusion. The fluid extract is preferable. The decoction is made by steeping 1 t. bark into 1 C. boiling water for ½ hr. Dose, 1 or 2 C. daily. An infusion is made by steeping ½ oz. bark in 1 pt. boiling water. Dose, 1 T. or as required.

CRANESBILL *(Geranium Maculatum)*

The name Cranesbill refers to the long beak-like projection on the seed. It is also known as alum root, which refers to its styptic properties.

Indigenous, cranesbill grows throughout the U.S. It is no relation to the geraniums of our gardens, which belong to the genus *pelargonium*.

The ROOT is the official part. It should be collected in the autumn. It has an astringent taste without bitterness or other unpleasant flavor. Water and alcohol extracts its virtues.

Cranesbill is considered a popular Indian remedy for various disorders.

Cranesbill is considered one of our most powerful astringents with pleasant tonic properties. The absence of unpleasant taste and all other offensive qualities and its soothing influence renders it peculiarly serviceable in cases of infants or of persons with very delicate stomachs, especially if boiled in milk with a little sugar.

Its chief influence is manifested throughout the alvine mucous membrane.

It is not so strong as oak bark or catechu but is a more powerful astringent than witch hazel. It is a tonic to the whole system; strengthens and invigorates stomach, kidneys, and the whole viscera.

Diarrhea, chronic dysentery, cholera infantum in the latter stages, excessive discharges in typhoid fever, sore mouth or gums, spongy gums, catarrhal ophthalmia, mercurial salivation are some of the diseases in which it is most commonly used to advantage. It is also useful in incontinence of urine.

As an application to indolent ulcers, an injection in gleet and leucorrhea, a gargle in relaxation of the uvula and aphthous ulceration of the throat, or throat irritation, it answers the same purpose as foreign remedies of the same character.

In gastric ulcer combine with golden seal.

A serviceable injection for leucorrhea is made by combining ½ oz. ea. of cranesbill and bethroot. Crush the roots and pour on 1 pt. boiling water. Cover until cool enough to use. Inject the clear liquid only. Repeat twice daily. Also good to use for mennorrhagia.

As a styptic, it is excellent for hemorrhages from the nose, lungs, stomach, bowels, or uterus. The Fl. X. may be used for internal or external bleeding.

Cranesbill can be used internally, externally, as injection, or as a wash wherever needed. It may be taken in substance, decoction, tincture, infusion, or Fl X. The dose of the powder is 20 to 30 gr. The decoction is made by boiling 1 oz. root in 1½ pts. water to 1 pt. Dose is 1 to 2 fl. oz. Dose of the Fl X is ½ to 1 Dr. The simple infusion is made by steeping 1 t. crushed root in 1 C. boiling water for ½ hr. Drink cold 1 or 2 C. daily.

CULVERS ROOT (Leptandra Virginica)

Culvers root is a native of the U.S. and grows throughout the country. The best (medicinally) is grown where there is limestone.

The ROOT, which is the part used, is gathered in the fall of the 2nd year. The taste is bitter and yields its active properties to boiling water.

Culvers rt. ranks high as a mild, persistent and reliable relaxant to the liver. Its influence is, to a very large extent, manifested upon the liver tubuli; it therefore assists the secretion of

41

bile but not the excretion through the gall ducts. It can be used internally or externally.

The cathartic action is slow. Large doses must be given if a physic is desired. Preparation of the green root in decoction is more cathartic than the dry.

While culvers rt. is not a pure cathartic, its influence being of a relaxing nature, it will be manifested upon the whole alvine mucous membrane; relaxing and dislodging viscid alvine accumulations.

If nauseating to the stomach, make a pad of equal parts of culver rt. and cayenne and use it externally over the liver. Moisten occasionally with the Fl. X or the tincture. An equal portion of bitter root may also be added.

Culvers rt. influences the small intestines somewhat definitely and has been much used in typhoid, diarrhea, and dysentery. Where the liver is not active enough in typhoid, typhus, bilious, remitting, rheumatic, and other fevers, it is invaluable.

In chronic constipation, in cases of hepatic failure, and in acute febrile conditions, although useful alone, it is best to combine culvers rt. with a cholagogue, and in jaundice this must always be the case, especially if the gall be somewhat solidified.

The following will influence both the secretory and excretory functions of the liver: simmer 1 oz. each culvers rt. and American mandrake in 1 qt. water for 20 min. Strain hot on ½ oz. ginger. Cover, strain, and take from 1 to 3 T. 3 or 4 times daily.

A good hepatic tonic is made as follows: all Fl. X, culvers rt. 4 Dr., golden seal ½ Dr., Gentian 15 drops, syrup ginger sufficient to make 4 oz. Take 1 t. doses from 1 to 4 times daily.

In torpor or congestion of the liver, the following may be taken in capsules once or twice a day: Mix together 1 Gr. each culvers rt. and American mandrake and ½ gr. each of bitter rt. and cayenne.

The Fl. X has been much used in recent years and may be taken in doses of ½ to 1 fl. Dr. The decoction is made by steeping 1 heaping t. of the root cut in small pieces into 1 C. boiling water for ½ hr. Drink 1 C. during a day. Doses of the powder is ¼ to 1 Dr. or 15 to 20 Gr.

DANDELION (*Taraxacum Officinale*)
The common name of this plant was derived from the fan-

cied resemblance of its leaves to the teeth of a lion.

A native of the Old World, it is now abundant in this country. It shows itself in the beginning of spring and continues to appear until near the close of summer. The leaves, when young, are not unpleasant to the taste, and are sometimes used as a salad. When older, they are medicinal. The U.S. Pharmacopea recognizes only the ROOT, which is by far the most efficacious part of the plant. It should be fully grown and collected fresh, as it is then most active, but the dug-up root, if dried with care, can be used in the succeeding winter. It is without smell but has a bitterish, herbaceous taste. Its active properties are yielded to water by boiling. The blossoms have been used by the Europeans for wine, and the seeds are eaten extensively by the birds.

An old time remedy, dandelion has been much employed medicinally in Germany and is now very popular in this country. It is thought to have a specific action upon the liver. It influences the liver in both its secreting and excreting function.

The diseases to which it appears to be especially applicable are those connected with derangement of the hepatic system and of the digestive organs generally, such as torpid liver, congestion and chronic inflammation of the liver and spleen, indigestion, constipation, jaundice, dropsy and in cases of suspended or deficient biliary secretion or in dropsical affections dependent on obstruction of the abdominal viscera. It is capable of doing much good. Also useful in dyspepsia, gout, and rheumatism.

An irritable condition of the stomach and bowels and the existence of acute inflammation contra-indicate its use.

A pleasant way of taking dandelion is as a substitute for coffee. The roasted roots are ground and used as ordinary coffee, tasting much like the regular coffee. This contains most of the beneficial medicinal properties.

A decoction of the roots or leaves in white wine is very effectual in opening and cleansing obstruction in the liver, gall, and spleen diseases that arise from such as jaundice, etc. It also opens urine passages. Dandelion will give great relief in cachexy from progressive consumption.

Dandelion is the best source of vit. A and also contains a liberal supply of vit. B 1, C, and G. Vit. A is known to help to prevent and dissolve stones and gravel. It is recommended that older people, in particular, should take it as a food to prevent the formation of stones.

Dandelion can be chopped raw and used to top sour cream, on baked potatoes, in soups and potato salad.

Medicinally it is usually given in the form of extract or decoction; 2 oz. of the fresh root or 1 oz. of the dried, bruised, or sliced may be boiled with 1 pt. water down to ½ pt. or 2 fl. oz. of the preparation taken twice or 3 times daily.

Aromatics may be added if there is a tendency to griping or flatulence.

ECHINACEA *(Echinacea Angustifolia)*

A native of the U.S., growing mostly on the Western prairies.

The ROOT is the part used. It has thick black roots with a pungent taste and no odor. It is largely used in impurities of the blood as boils, carbuncles, gangrene, puerperal septicemia, and tuberculosis; it is used both internally and externally. For tuberculosis, elecampane root may be added.

For boils and carbuncles, apply an external application of equal parts echinacea and ground pine, at the same time taking internally equal parts FE echinacea and simple syrup. Dose: 1 Dr. 3 to 6 times daily.

For fermentative dyspepsia, typhoid, and other fevers, add ½ to 1 Dr. FE to other remedies for good results.

In puerperal septicemia take ½ to 1 t. every 4 hours.

For black tongue, indicating low septic conditions, mix FE echinacea 1 Dr. or more in 4 oz. distilled water; take 1 Dr. every 3 hrs.

In erysypelis and in poison ivy poisoning, apply Fl. X for almost instant relief.

As a blood purifier, mix (all FE) 2 Dr. ea. of echinacea, Jamaica sarsaparilla and burdock rt., 1 Dr. each false bittersweet and juniper berries and 8 oz. simple syrup. Dose 1 t. or more 3 times daily.

A simple infusion is made as follows: steep 1 t. granulated root in 1 C. boiling water ½ hr. Strain and take 1 T. 3 to 6 times daily.

ELECAMPANE *(Inula Helenium)*

This plant is a native of Europe where it is cultivated for

medical use. It has now become naturalized in some parts of this country.

The ROOT is the official part, and should be dug up in autumn, in the 2nd year of its growth. When older, it is apt to be stringy and woody.

The taste is aromatic and bitter; the odor is slightly camphorous and, especially in the dried root, agreeably aromatic. Its medical virtues are extracted by alcohol and water; the former being most strongly impregnated with its bitterness and pungency.

By the ancients it was much employed, especially in the complaints peculiar to females and is still used in cases of retained or suppressed menses.

From a belief in its deobstruent and diuretic virtues, it was formerly prescribed in chronic engorgements of the abdominal viscera and the dropsy to which they so often give rise.

It is now considered valuable in chronic diseases of the lungs, coughs, asthma, bronchitis, and all chest troubles, especially with weakness of the digestive organs and with general debility. It is warming and strengthening to the lungs while at the same time it promotes the expectoration of viscid mucus. It is especially recommended in tuberculosis of the lungs. It is claimed that a combination of elecampane and echinacea is very useful in tuberculosis.

It has been highly recommended both as an internal and external remedy in tetter, psora, and other diseases of the skin. It is because of this that elecampane is also called scabwort.

Elecampane is also a warming, strengthening, cleansing tonic remedy to the mucous membrane, especially the gastric, alvine, and pulmonary membranes, and is of excellent use in catarrhal conditions of the bronchi and dyspepsia. It is better suited to chronic than acute conditions.

It is an excellent addition to cough syrups. An infusion of the root, sweetened with honey, will be found useful in whooping cough, although the infusion of thyme is most frequently used for this trouble.

The usual methods of using are in powder or decoction. The dose of the powder is a scruple to a drachm. The decoction may be prepared by boiling ½ oz. root in 1 pt. water and taken in doses of 1 or 2 fl. oz.

In hot infusion, its stimulating power gives a good outward circulation.

(RED) SLIPPERY ELM *(Ulmus Fulva)*

(Red) slippery elm was the food and medicine of the pioneers and the American Indians.

Indigenous to the U.S., it grows north of the Carolinas but is most abundant west of the Allegheny Mountains.

The INNER BARK is the part used in medicine. It has a peculiar sweetish, but not unpleasant, odor, and a highly mucilaginous taste when chewed. By grinding, it is reduced to a light, grayish fawn-colored powder. It abounds in mucilaginous matter, which it readily imparts to water.

Red elm is one of the finest and most valuable remedies in the herbal world and should be in every home; there is nothing in this world to equal it. It is one of the best for internal or external use wherever there is an irritation or inflamed condition.

It is especially recommended in diseases and inflammatory conditions of the urinary organs, the stomach, lungs, intestines, and in dysentery, diarrhea, constipation, or cholera infantum used both orally and in rectal injection. It lubricates and soothes.

It is very useful in leprous and herpetic eruptions, tetters, and in all skin diseases, inflammations, and irritations, purulent ophthalmia, chilblains, ulcers, wounds, burns, boils, carbuncles, abscesses, etc. used externally as a poultice. It soothes the part, disperses the inflammation, draws out the impurities, and heals quickly. Also during the scaling process in scarletina and measles and at times in typhoid fever. Mix the coarse powder with hot or boiling water and apply as hot as convenient, change as often as required.

For an obstinate boil, mix 3 parts powdered red elm and 1 part powdered lobelia. A wash with red elm is good for sores on any part of the body. For burns, scaled and abraded skin, add to linseed oil. Keep well covered. There is nothing better.

Inflammation in the bowels of infants or adults has been cured with using an injection of an infusion of 1 oz. powdered bark in 1 pt. boiling water, stirring frequently. When at proper temperature, inject into the bowels.

Red elm is fully as nutritious as oatmeal. We are told that

it has proved sufficient for the support of life in the absence of other food. The instance of a soldier is reported who lived for 10 days in the woods on this bark and sassafras. The Indians are said to resort to it for nutriment in emergencies.

A pleasant drink may be made by stirring the powder in hot water, with which it forms a mucilage, more or less thick, according to the proportion added.

Red elm GRUEL is perhaps the most useful of foods.

In debilitated conditions of the stomach, when all food is rejected, it is frequently found that the gruel will be gratefully received. (Note—The author can heartily recommend this gruel. When my mother, who had cancer, could keep nothing on her stomach and was unable to take solid food, she was able to retain elm gruel. She took it through a baby bottle. Another relative who had painter's colic said nothing helped him like this gruel.)

The gruel is made as follows: mix 1½ t. powdered bark and 1 t. sugar, or more if desired, to a paste with cold water. Heat 1 C. milk to the boiling point and stir in the elm paste, continue on a low heat for a few seconds. Take off the stove, beat with an egg beater or blender to take out the lumps. Add a dash of powdered cinnamon or nutmeg, if desired. Drink warm, as much as desired. It is very soothing and healing to inflamed surfaces and is very strengthening.

In weakness, inflammation of the stomach, bleeding of the lungs, consumption, asthma, bronchitis, pneumonia, gastritis, nephritis, gastric ulcer, pyloric inflammation or ulceration, calculus, scalding urine, etc., take red elm gruel.

For weaning infants, the gruel may be thinned with added milk or water. It will soothe the baby's stomach, and baby will be fed at the same time.

For a good healing food drink, beat 1 egg with 1 t. powdered red elm. Pour on 1 C. boiling milk. Stir and sweeten to taste.

Red elm gruel is considered a specific in ulcerated stomach.

It is soothing to the mucous membrane wherever needed, especially in croup and diphtheria after the false membrane has been cleaned out and the throat is quite raw.

Red Elm is also used in the formation of lozenges and suppositories. The lozenges are excellent for coughs due to colds and to relieve an irritated pharynx. The suppositories are important in treating inflammation of the ovaries, vagina, uterine weakness, pruritis, leucorrhea or growths.

An excellent remedy for an infected sore is as follows: Add 1 t. fine brown sugar and 1½ t. powdered elm bark to the white of an egg. Mix but do not beat. Cover the sore with this coating. Change every 15 min.

MAIDENHAIR FERN (*Adiantum Pedatum*)

Also called Northern and American Maidenhair. *Adiantum Capillus-Veneris* is called Southern Maidenhair.

The *Collier Dictionary* says *adiantum* is a Greek word meaning "unwetted." This fern is said to have the property of repelling moisture, and if placed under water, when removed, will be found to be perfectly dry.

In Roman mythology, it was believed to be the hair of Venus, goddess of love and beauty, who, when she arose from the sea, had dry hair. Because of this, lotions made of maidenhair have been made up to keep the hair from going out of curl on damp days.

Maidenhair fern grows wild throughout the U.S. mostly in deep woods. The leaves are somewhat bitter and slightly aromatic. They part with their medical virtues upon being immersed in boiling water.

Maidenhair influences the mucous membrane throughout the whole system. In Europe it is used largely as a cough medicine, and is very well-known there under the name of "*Sirop de Capillare*." A strong decoction will soothe bronchial irritation, colds, coughs, especially irritable coughs, throat affections, all pulmonary troubles, nasal congestion, catarrh, and hoarseness. It can be taken freely.

An addition of white poplar is good for the urinary tract. An addition of uva ursi will be soothing to the kidneys, bladder, uterus, and the urethra. It will relieve cystic catarrh and scalding urine. An addition of comfrey root and horehound will be a favorable influence on the bronchi. An addition of golden seal or gentian will greatly benefit the alvine canal.

Maidenhair has also been used as a hair tonic. It is said that if ashes of the fern are mixed with olive oil and vinegar, this will prevent premature baldness or loss of hair from disease.

It may be used in infusion or decoction; 1 oz. of the herb to 1 pt. water, taking ½ pt. to 1 pint a day in wine-glassful doses. Honey or sugar may be added, if desired.

MALE FERN *(Aspidium Filix Mas)*

Indigenous and growing in the shady pine forests over most of the U.S.

The ROOT is the part used. The proper time for collecting the root is during the summer when it abounds more in the active principles than at any other season. It should be carefully prepared as it deteriorates rapidly when kept and in about 2 years becomes entirely inert. In powdering the root, only the internal portion should be preserved. The dried root has a peculiar but feeble odor and a sweetish, bitter, astringent, nauseous taste.

The male fern is a famous remedy used for the expulsion of all kinds of worms, especially tape worms.

The widow of a Swiss surgeon, Madam Nouffer, attained such fame in treating tapeworm that the King of France purchased the secret of her treatment and published it in 1775. The treatment was to give a free dose of the powdered male fern, followed in 2 or 3 hours by an active cathartic, repeating the dose in 2 or 3 days until the worm was passed. European physicians used this article most successfully after this. It is claimed, however, that a German physician had used the male fern in a similar manner before Madam Nouffer's secret was known.

It is claimed that the medicine acts specifically against the worms which it speedily destroys, and this favors its expulsion from the body without producing any severe or unpleasant symptoms.

The medicine may be given in powder or in fluid extract. The dose of the powder is 1 to 3 dr. to be given in the form of electuary or emulsion and repeated morning and evening for 1 or 2 days successively. Or the powder may be taken in capsules, in honey, or in infusion. The emulsion is made as a thick mucilage of gum arabic and water adding ½ to 1 dr. of powder. It should be taken on an empty stomach in the morning, repeating if necessary in 2 or 3 days. Follow with a purge of senna with ginger or of butternut bark, if desired. The dose of the fluid X is from 12 to 24 gr. The decoction is used in the proportion of 1 oz. root to 1 pt. water.

The oil extracted from the root is taken in doses of 30 drops in emulsion or capsules, or in warm water night and morning.

A good method for giving children male fern is as follows: take equal parts of the fluid extract and glycerine, place the bottle in warm water to get them well mixed, shake well, and give as follows: 4–7 years, 6 drops in jam; 7–12 years, 12 drops in jam, and over 12 years, 1 to 2 t. in ½ C. cold tea about 6 A.M. on an empty stomach.

For those over 12 years, follow with 2 oz. Senna, ½ oz. mt. flax, and 1 large lemon, sliced. Cover with 2 pts. boiling water and let steep ½ hr. Give ½ pt. at 8 A.M., breakfast at 9 A.M. Repeat once a week for 3 or 4 weeks.

The author had tapeworms as a child. The M.D. ordered a tea made of pumpkin seeds, fasting that day. To my recollection, that took care of the worms quite thoroughly.

FIGWORT (*Scrophularia Nodosa*)

Although a native of Europe, figwort is now growing in the northern section of the U.S. It is also called scrofula plant because its medicinal virtues are said to be particularly directed to this condition. The plant is distinguished by its knotty roots.

The LEAVES, ROOTS, and the HERB are used and yield their virtues to water and alcohol. The leaves, when fresh, have a rank fetid odor and a bitter somewhat acrid taste; but these properties are diminished by drying. Water extracts their virtues, forming a reddish infusion.

They influence the secernents and tone the pelvic organs and the kidneys, increasing the quantity of urine.

The leaves and herb, applied as a poultice, ointment, or fomentation, are useful in piles, scrofula, painful tumors, ulcers, skin diseases, sores, cutaneous eruptions, abscesses, sprains, swellings, inflammations and bruises. Also taken internally in infusion of 1 oz. leaves to 1 pt. boiling water in ½ wine-glassful doses.

In skin diseases, the following will be a good combination: 2 oz. figwort and 1 oz. each of yellow dock rt. and queens delight rt. Simmer in 2 qts. water down to 2½ pts. and take 3 T. 3 or 4 times daily.

Where there is weakness of the generative organs and irregular menstruation, it will be a soothing tonic.

BLUE FLAG (*Iris Versicolor*)

The blue flag is found in all parts of the U.S. The ROOT is the medicinal portion. The flowers form a fine blue infusion which serves as a test of acids and alkalies.

The root in the green state is somewhat acrid, but when dried this is lost and the virtues of the root is unimpaired. It imparts its virtue to boiling water or alcohol. It is said to be held in much esteem by the southern Indians.

Its influence extends through the secernants, influencing the whole glandular and lymphatic system stimulating the flow of saliva and bile.

It is useful in impurity of the blood, constipation especially if chronic, rheumatism especially if chronic, dropsy, skin diseases, mercurial cachexis, leuchorrhea, chronic liver troubles, sluggish circulation, and it has quite a reputation in the treatment of syphilis, secondary syphilis, scrofula, and other venereal diseases. Its best advantage is in chronic and torpid conditions.

Cold preparations quite freely influence the liver, gall ducts, and bowels. Large doses are sometimes nauseating.

It is said to give good results in goitre.

As a laxative, only small doses are taken, the Fl. X being often used for this purpose.

In hot infusion, blue flag stimulates a good free outward circulation.

As an alterative for glandular and skin troubles, the following is recommended: all FE, 2 Dr. ea. dandelion, Jamaica sarsaparilla, yellow dock and burdock seeds, 20 drops FE prickly ash and 4 oz. of simple syrup. Dose—1 to 3 times daily.

It is claimed the following has been used successfully in uterine fibroids: all FE, 6 Dr. blue flag, 4 Dr. golden seal, 5 Dr. balmony, 2 Dr. prickly ash and 16 oz. of simple syrup.

Blue flag may be taken in substance, decoction, or tincture. The dose of the dried root is from 10 to 20 gr. The Fl X may be used for all the general purposes of the root.

Where there are irritable conditions, blue flag is NOT to be used.

AMERICAN GENTIAN *(Gentiana Catesbaei)*

Indigenous, the American or blue gentian grows in the grassy swamps and meadows of North and South Carolina.

The dried root has at first a mucilaginous and sweetish taste, which is soon succeeded by an intense bitterness, approaching nearly to that of the official gentian. Alcohol and water extract its virtues. The tincture and decoction are even more bitter than the root in substance.

This gentian is recognized by the medical profession as having similar medical properties to the foreign gentian *(Gentiana Lutea)*, and may be used as a substitute for it in the same doses and preparations.

Used principally in dyspepsia and cases of stomachic and general debility.

May be taken in powder 15 or 30 gr. or substituted for foreign gentian in the preparation of the official Fl. X, infusion, wine, and tincture.

For other uses see Foreign Gentian.

GOLDEN SEAL *(Hydrastis Canadensis)*

It is claimed the American Indians first used this plant as a tonic. It is also called yellow root because the root is of a beautiful yellow color and used by the Indians as a dye.

It is found in the woods in the U.S. The ROOT must, however, be 4 years old before taking it up for use. It is intensely bitter, somewhat unpleasant to the taste and has a most disagreeable odor. It is, however, most reliable.

Golden seal has been well-named the "king of tonics" to the mucous membrane. It has been a popular and useful remedy since 1820. It is a positive and permanent stimulating tonic. Its influence, though primarily applicable to debilitated conditions of the mucous membrane, extends to all parts of the body wherever it may be required.

It is eligible for combination with almost any other remedies where a tonic is needed. It can be made to especially influence the stomach, bowels, respiratory organs, urinary tract, or generative organs by combining it with remedies which especially influence these parts.

Combined with squaw vine *(mitchella)* its influence will quickly manifest itself upon the organs of generation; with butternut, it is a powerful intestinal tonic; combined with gravel root, the kidneys will soon feel its influence, and with comfrey, it gives tone and vigor to the respiratory organs.

It is very useful in the vomiting of pregnancy.

Golden seal is one of the very few remedies which will tone and sustain the venous circulation. Its special function with the liver is its tonic relief to the portal circulation; hence its action upon the right side or the venous side of the heart. With hepatics, golden seal will influence both the secreting and excreting functions of the liver.

It is extremely useful in disordered states of the digestive apparatus, in dyspepsia, gastric catarrh, gastric irritation, and gastric ulceration. It will improve the appetite and aid digestion. In cases where the gastric membrane is clogged with congestion or catarrhal mucus, in weak or debilitated stomach, especially where there is nervous disturbance, take golden seal in small and frequent doses. It will also assist in overcoming constipation with hard dry stools.

In female troubles it is unexcelled. Witch hazel may be added as required. The infusion is a most efficient vaginal douche in leucorrhea, and can be used daily in uterine ulceration. Also a good wash for inflamed or sore eyes and ulcers in the mouth.

A very fine golden seal tonic is made by boiling together 16 oz. golden seal, 100 oz. water, and 28 oz. glycerine down to 114 oz. Strain and bottle.

A very fine tonic that will stimulate, sustain, and tone the spinal nerves is made as follows: infuse 1 oz. golden seal, ¾ oz. hops, and ½ oz. skullcap in 1½ pts. boiling water. Cover till nearly cold. Strain and take freely from a wine-glassful 3 times daily. This may also be compounded in powder form and filled into #4 capsules and taken 2 or 3 capsules every 2 hrs.

In the eruptive diseases such as smallpox, measles, etc., where there is much itching and burning of the skin, and in scarlatina to prevent the scales spreading from the patient, wash with FE golden seal 1 oz. and 9 oz. linseed oil. It will bring relief.

A decoction of golden seal used as a wash in smallpox will allay the itching, relieve the nervous system, and so tone the new cuticle under the postules as to greatly lessen the danger of pitting. It may be used several times a day upon the face and hands. Follow each application with a light dressing of sweet oil.

Adding glycerine forms a good wash in gonorrhea.

Golden seal will give good service in erysipelas, ophthalmia, sore mouth and throat, eruptive and syphilitic sores.

An infusion of golden seal may be used daily for ulceration. It may be snuffed up the nostrils for nasal congestion or catarrh.

In grandular opthalmia, with ulceration of the cornea, the following will be of decided value; infuse 1 oz. golden seal, ¼ oz. lobelia herb, 20 gr. cayenne in 1 pt. boiling water. Cover till almost cold. Strain and use as a wash. In some cases it may be preferable to use the powdered gum myrrh in place of the cayenne.

Golden seal is one of the finest remedies in powder form for the treatment of irritable chancres and buboes and in treating lip ulcers in syphilis. Used as follows it will give every satisfaction: all in powder; 4 dr. golden seal, 1 Dr. myrrh, 5 gr. cayenne. Rub well in mortar and fill the ulcer several times a day.

The decoction, fluid extract, or tincture is a good local application for ringworms.

In purchasing the fluid extract, there are 2 kinds offered for sale: the ordinary fluid extract and the colorless. For washes and injections, the colorless preparation would prevent the staining of the linen, yet for general use it is inferior and does not contain all the therapeutic value of the root.

Golden seal can be used in infusion, decoction, fluid extract, or substance. The fluid extract has been much used in recent years but the fresh root is preferred.

OREGON GRAPE *(Berberis Aquifolium)*

Also known as holly-leaved barberry, it grows principally in California. The taste is bitter, and the plant has no odor.

Oregon grape ROOT is of much value in impurities of the blood and most skin diseases, particularly of the chafy and scaly kind, in eczema, and in scrofulous conditions.

Excellent in the treatment of syphilis cases and other blood diseases affecting the genitals.

Oregon grape's influence to the alvine mucous membrane is mildly cathartic. In chronic constipation, combine with cascara sagrada for good results.

As a tonic hepatic, it influences the liver, particularly in chronic conditions.

In tubercular trachoma use, all FE, 4 Dr. each Oregon grape

and bugle weed, 2 Dr. prickly ash bark and 4 oz. queen's delight—dose 1 t. 3 times daily.

A simple infusion is made by steeping 1 t. root in 1 C. boiling water. Strain and take 1 T. 4 times daily.

Oregon grape may be substituted for golden seal.

GRAVEL ROOT *(Eupatorium Purpureum)*

Gravel root grows in low grounds from Canada to Virginia across the U.S.

The ROOT is the official portion. It has a bitter, aromatic, and astringent taste, and its virtues yield to water by decoction or alcohol.

Gravel root is one of our best herbs in many urinary troubles. It influences the kidneys, bladder, and uterus; relaxes and gently stimulates and tones the pelvic viscera. It has become popular because of its beneficial influence in deposits of brick dust and gravel. It is claimed, by some, that bad cases of gravel have been cured by this plant alone. Some claim that dropsy has been cured by this plant.

In febrile conditions with scanty urine, either with or without the brick dust deposits, it is a very fine remedy. In bloody urine, painful or scalding micturation, prostatic, especially irritated prostatic troubles, irritated urinary tract, in spermatorrhea, acute and chronic gonorrhea, urethral, uterine and vaginal irritations, aching back and general pelvic weakness, it is a valuable remedy. Large doses, by its influence in toning the mucous membrane, cause a casting off of sediments that may have settled on the surfaces. It is often noted that after using gravel root, quite a deposit is seen in the urine. It is because of its use in gravel that the common name of gravel root has been given to it.

It is very soothing to the kidneys and gently toning by relief of irritation and increasing the flow of urine. In these respects it is one of the most reliable remedies.

By increasing the elimination of solids in the urine, it is at times useful in acute rheumatism. In the depressed state of typhoid it should be combined with stimulating remedies such as cayenne and juniper.

A good combination in pelvic troubles is made by simmering 1½ oz. gravel rt., 1 oz. golden seal, 1 oz. squaw vine *(mitchella)* in 2½ pts. water for 20 min. Strain and take 3 T. 3 times daily. This is also a nervine tonic.

In the suppression of the menses, it is splendid and always safe. It needs to be given in large quantities, but always leaves a toned condition.

GUAIACUM *(Guaiacum Officinale)*

This is a tropical tree native to the W. Indies, with some growing in So. California and So. Florida. The common name given to it, *lignum vitae,* means "wood of life," evidently referring to its medicinal properties.

All parts of the tree possess medicinal properties, but the WOOD and the CONCRETE JUICE (gum resin) only are official. The bark, considered much more efficacious than the wood, is not available.

Guaiacum wood is imported from Haiti, Jamaica, and other W. Indies Islands in the shape of logs. These are used for the fabrication of various instruments and utensils for which the wood is well adapted by its extreme hardness and density. It is kept by druggists only in the state of chips or raspings which they obtain from the turners.

The wood is almost without smell unless rubbed or heated, when it then becomes odorous. When burnt, it emits an agreeable odor. It is bitterish and slightly pungent and requires to be chewed for some time before the taste is developed. Its medicinal properties are probably dependent on the guaiac with which it is impregnated. It yields its virtues but partially to water. Alcohol is the best solvent.

Gum guaiacum or guaiac is the concrete juice of the tree obtained by spontaneous exudation or by incisions made into the trunk. There are also other methods. Guaiac is brought to the market from the West Indies. It is readily pulverized. Though commonly called gum guaiac and till recently considered a gum resin, it has been ascertained to be a substance neither containing nor consisting of gum or resin. It is therefore properly designated by the simple title, guaiacum. Both the WOOD and the GUM RESIN are used by botanic practitioners.

The wood is largely used in the manufacture of blood purifiers, often combined with sarsaparilla.

Guaiacum is most beneficial in mercurial cachexia, secondary syphilis, venereal rheumatism especially chronic rheumatism, gout, scrofulous affections, impurities of the blood, cutaneous eruptions, eczema, and protracted diseases dependent on a depraved or debilitated condition of the system. A decoction is preferred in combination with compound decoction of sarsaparilla. The wood, however, seems to be favored in these complaints. It is said to be useful in amenorrhoea.

It influences the digestive, urinary, and genital organs, stimulates the circulation, and induces a good capillary flow. It is best suited to languid and depressed conditions of the mucous membranes and a clogged condition of the secernents.

The gum resin is not a good remedy to use in irritated or inflamed conditions as it is too stimulating. In large doses, it purges.

The following is considered effective in the treatment of rheumatism: 1 dr. powdered gum guaiacum, 2 Dr. powdered rhubarb, 1 oz. each cream of tartar, and finely powdered nutmeg. Mix with 1# honey. Take 2 large spoonfuls night and morning.

The Dominion Herbal College claims excellent results in rheumatism from the following: all in powder: 1 oz. of each gum guaiacum, cayenne, sulphur, turkey rhubarb. Mix and fill #1 capsules and take 4 of the capsules 2 or 3 times daily.

A simple decoction of the wood is prepared by boiling 1 oz. in 1½ pts. water down to 1 pt., the whole of which is taken during 24 hrs.

The gum is taken in substance or tincture. The dose of the powder is from 10 to 30 gr. which may be taken in pills or mixed with sugar and taken in capsules or in an emulsion made with gum arabic, sugar, and water. An objection to the powder is that it quickly aggregates. The resin does not readily combine with other remedies.

The simple infusion of the wood is made by steeping 1 oz. in 1 pt. boiling water, 1 wine-glassful to be taken.

Cold doses are usually best for chronic diseases.

HEMLOCK SPRUCE (*Abies Canadensis*)

This is the hemlock spruce of the U.S., growing mostly in the elevated or mountainous regions.

The bark is much used for tanning purposes. By incising the bark, the tree yields a heavy black pitch or hemlock gum only used as an ingredient in plasters. It is usually incorporated with oils.

The INNER BARK is frequently used in composition powders. It is rarely used alone. It is often used in infusion as a wash in leucorrhea, buboes, ulcers, especially rectal ulcers, hemorrhoids, hemorrhage, and diarrhea.

It makes an excellent gargle for sore mouth and spongy gums.

A good suppository is made for hemorrhoids as follows; all in powder, 2 oz. hemlock spruce, 1 oz. ea. golden seal, wheat flour, boracic acid, and bayberry bark. Mix together and add sufficient glycerine to form suppositories of the size desired. Insert one at night. Rectal pain will be quickly relieved.

The LEAVES are more stimulating and less astringent. In hot infusion they will relieve colds and dysmenorrhoea. Used in hot fomentation, it is valuable for sprains, rheumatism, and inflammations. DO NOT USE if constipated.

The OIL of hemlock is obtained from the LEAVES and is more stimulating. It is useful as an addition to liniments. It is NOT taken internally.

GARDEN HOLLYHOCK *(Althea Rosea)*

This plant grows in gardens all over the U.S. Its name is derived from *altheao*—meaning "to cure."

The WHOLE PLANT is used. The medicinal properties of the garden hollyhock is similar to the marshmallow, it is often substituted for it and may be used for the same general purposes.

It is not quite as mucilaginous as the marshmallow, but has a more pronounced influence upon the kidneys, bladder, and the whole urinary organs.

In chest troubles, where irritated surfaces need an emollient and demulcent, it is very soothing to the mucous membrane.

In inflammation of the bladder, tenderness or sensitive conditions of the prostate or neck of the bladder, it will be found excellent.

In gonorrhea, the following combination is recommended: golden seal, witch hazel, hollyhock or marshmallow. The golden seal should be used in excess in the primary stage and the witch hazel should be used in excess subsequently. In irritable coughs and colds add spikenard and wild cherry and in diabetes, add false bittersweet.

Excellent used as a gargle in swollen tonsils and in relaxation of the uvula.

HOPS (*Humulus Lupulus*)

This is the common or European hops, now widely naturalized and growing wild in many places in the U.S. Most of the hops consumed in the U.S. are supplied from New England where it is extensively cultivated. It is claimed the English hops are superior to all others.

Besides being important in brewing beer, ale, and porter it is of some ornamental value. The part used in preparation of malt liquors and in medicine is the FRUIT or STROBILES.

Though brittle when quite dry, they are pulverized with great difficulty. Their odor is strong, peculiar, somewhat narcotic, and fragrant; their taste is very bitter, aromatic, and slightly astringent. Their aroma, bitterness, and astringency are imparted to boiling water by decoction, but the aroma is dissipated by long boiling. A better solvent is diluted alcohol.

The activity of hops depends upon a substance secreted by the scales and in the dried fruit existing upon their surface in the form of a fine powder. This substance is called LUPULIN. It is considered official. It is preferable to the hops because of its convenience. The virtues of the lupulin probably reside in the volatile oil and bitter principle, which are readily imparted to alcohol. By boiling in water the bitterness is extracted, but the aroma is partially driven off.

Hops are tonic and moderately narcotic, and have been highly recommended in diseases of general or local debility associated with morbid insomnia or other nervous derangements, sleeplessness, hysteria, and delirium. They have a most soothing effect and will frequently promote sleep in overwrought conditions. An infusion of 1 oz. to 1 pt. boiling water may be taken in doses of 2 or 3 T. every 1, 2, or 3 hours as needed. They have some tendency to relieve pain, and may be used for these purposes in cases where opiates, from their tendency to constipate, or other causes, are inadmissable.

The Dominion College claims the FLOWERS are a fine stimulating and relaxing nervine of great powers.

They claim the hops pillow has been used from early days in insomnia and is very effective. Stuffing a pillow with hops and using as an ordinary pillow will soothe and quiet the whole nervous system, allay restlessness, and produce sleep in cases of nervous derangements. Others claim the hops should be moistened with alcohol in order to prevent their rustling noise and to bring out the active principle.

The complaints in which hops have been found useful are dyspepsia, nervous tremors, delirium of drunkards, and in dysmenorrhoea.

The extract is advantageous in allaying the pain of articular rheumatism and neuralgia when taken internally or as a hot fomentation applied on the parts affected.

Fomentations with hops and a poultice made by mixing them with some emollient adhesive substance are often beneficial in local pains and swellings, bruises, inflammations, rheumatism, neuralgia, boils, and gatherings. It is often used alone, and may be combined with camomile, poppy heads, or ragwort.

An ointment of the powder with lard is recommended as an application to sores, the pain of which it relieves when other means have failed.

Hops also has a reputation in Calculi, are useful in some liver troubles and jaundice, relieving the secernents because of a favorable alterative property. They have a relaxing influence upon the liver and gall duct and are very gently laxative to the bowels.

For worms, take ½ to 1 pt. decoction made of 1 oz. to the pint, in the morning.

Hops are useful in excessive sexual desire, pruritis, and painful erections in gonorrhea.

Hops may be added to cough syrups for irritable coughs.

A flannel bag filled with hops and heated will often relieve toothache and neuralgia.

Hops may be taken in substance, infusion, tincture, or extract.

An infusion is prepared from 1 oz. to 1 pt. boiling water, taken in doses of 2 fl. oz. 3 or 4 times daily. Good as a general tonic and sedative. The fluid extract and tincture are official.

All the effects of the preparation of hops may be obtained with greater certainty and convenience by the use of lupulin. The dose of this substance is from 6 to 12 gr., taken in the form of pills, which may be made by simply rubbing the powder in a warm mortar until it aquires the consistence of a ductile mass and then moulding into the proper shape.

Lupulin may be incorporated with poultices or formed into an ointment with lard and used externally for the same purpose as the hops themselves.

The tincture may be taken in ½ to 1 t. doses; the nerves will be quieted and no evil effects will follow such as are found after using opiates.

BLACK HOREHOUND *(Ballota Nigrum)*

Black horehound is a native of Europe, but is now naturalized in America. It has an unpleasant taste and the odor is disagreeable.

All that has been written for the white horehound also applies to the black horehound, except that in some conditions the black is preferable.

It is useful in amenorrhea, mennorhagia, dysmenorrhea, gravel, dropsy, coughs, hoarseness, bronchitis, consumption, and weak stomach.

It is considered almost a specific in biliousness, bilious colic, regurgitation of food and sour stomach.

Adding marshmallow, hyssop, and elecampane will enhance its use in lung affections and in troubles of the respiratory organs, especially if blood is expectorated. This will also act as an alterative and tonic to the mucous membranes; the mucous secretions will be influenced, irritated surfaces assisted, and the sharpness of the discharge corrected.

Adding motherwort will tone the uterine membrane.

It may be used in infusion, decoction, powder or pills.

WHITE OR COMMON HOREHOUND *(Marrubium Vulgare)*

This plant is a native of Europe, but has been naturalized in this country. Although cultivated in gardens, it now grows wild in many places.

The HERB has a strong, rather agreeable odor, which is diminished by drying and lost in keeping. The taste is bitter and aromatic. The bitterness is extracted by water and alcohol.

White horehound has been popular as a pectoral herb since the discovery of its healing qualities early in Greek and Roman history.

It is a tonic to the respiratory organs and to the stomach. In large doses, it is laxative.

It is one of the most popular of pectoral remedies. Taken cold it is exceedingly valuable in asthma, catarrh, especially wet catarrh, colds, and other chronic affections of the lungs attended with coughs and copious expectoration. Its expectorant properties assist in loosing phlegm.

A warm or hot infusion will relieve the hyperemic conditions of the lungs and congestion by promoting a good outward flow of blood.

It was once considered a valuable deobstruent and recommended in chronic hepatitis, jaundice, phthisis, and various general debility affections.

When the menstrual flow is obstructed by a recent cold, add a little ginger to the warm infusion. Sweeten with honey, if desired.

Excellent in children's cough, croup, and colds, it will sustain the vocal cords in congestion and hoarseness.

Horehound is considered excellent for those that have hard livers.

A candy is made as follows: boil 2 oz. dried herb in 1½ pts. water about ½ hr. Strain and add 3½# brown sugar. Boil until it reaches the proper degree of hardness. Pour into well greased flat trays. Mark into squares with a knife as it becomes cool enough to retain its shape. This is considered very useful in coughs, especially for older people and the asthmatic.

Syrup of horehound is made by boiling 1# sugar with the same quantity of leaves until syrupy.

The infusion is made by steeping 1 oz. of the herb in 1 pt. boiling water, adding honey, if desired. Take in wine-glassful doses.

Dose of the powder is from 30 gr. to 1 dr.

HORSERADISH *(Cochlearia Armoracia)*

Horseradish is a native of Europe, but is now cultivated in the U.S.

The ROOT, official in its fresh state, has a strong pungent odor when scraped or bruised and a hot biting, somewhat sweetish taste. Its virtues are imparted to water and alcohol, but destroyed by boiling. It may be kept for some time without material injury by being buried in sand in a cool place.

Horseradish will arouse a pleasant warmth in the stomach

when swallowed promoting the secretions, especially increasing the flow of urine.

Its chief use is as a condiment to promote appetite and invigorate digestion, but it is also occasionally employed as a medicine, particularly in dropsical complaints attended with an enfeebled condition of the digestive organs and of the system in general. It has been recommended in palsy and rheumatism, both as an internal and external remedy.

Horseradish is useful to the kidneys, jaundice, skin, circulation, will relieve the gall ducts, stimulate alvine action, tone the mucous membrane, and produce fullness of the pulse. Also in atonic dyspepsia with sluggish bile, and in gastric and intestinal catarrh.

For a torpid stomach and liver with constipation, try the following: ½ oz. ea. FE horseradish and tincture gentian, 1½ oz. FE dandelion, and 6 oz. syrup of orange. Dose 1 t. at mealtime.

The following is recommended for dropsy: pour 1 pt. boiling water on 1 oz. horseradish and ½ oz. crushed mustard seed. Cover until cold. Strain and take 2 to 3 T's., 3 times daily.

In scorbutic affections, horseradish is highly esteemed.

The fresh roots, as well as the leaves, will blister the skin if applied too long. Both can be used as a local application in neuralgia and relief can usually be obtained.

In hoarseness, use a syrup prepared from an infusion of horseradish and sugar and slowly swallow in 2 or 1 t. doses repeated as required. The root may be taken in doses of ½ dr. or more, grated or cut in small pieces.

The root in vinegar is a good table relish for a torpid stomach.

The freshly ground root blended with cider or wine vinegar will keep almost indefinitely. Adding grated raw carrot with a little mayonnaise is an excellent addition to any meal. Also fresh grated root added to ketchup, to taste, adds enjoyment to cooked fish, particularly shrimp, clams, and oysters.

HYSSOP (*Hyssopus Officinalis*)

Common hyssop is a native of Europe, where, just as in this country, it is cultivated in gardens. It is growing wild in many places over the U.S. today.

The FLOWERING TOPS and LEAVES are the official parts. The plant has an agreeable, aromatic odor and a warm, pungent, bitter taste. These they owe to an essential oil.

An infusion has been much used in cases of chronic catarrh, especially in old people and those of debilitated habit of body. It acts by facilitating the expectoration of the mucus which is too abundantly secreted.

Useful in chest diseases; colds, coughs, hoarseness, fevers, bronchial troubles, irritable tickling coughs, sore throat, lung troubles, also in kidney and liver affections.

The following will be useful in chest diseases: simmer 2 oz. hyssop in 1 qt. water for 15 min. Strain and make into syrup with honey. It will generally give relief in a very short time. Where the throat is sore, in addition to taking the above, gargle with the infusion a few times. The addition of sage will be helpful.

Also useful in removing discoloration from bruises or for a black eye. Place a handful of the herb on a cloth and soak in boiling water just enough to soak the herb through. Apply to the eye as a poultice.

In slow, lingering fevers, hyssop is a splendid remedy, especially with children. Simmer slowly, covered 1 oz. in 1 pt. of water for a few minutes, then allow to steep and keep warm. Take a wineglassful every hour. It will bring a gentle moisture to the skin, relieve the kidneys and bladder. Its gentle aperient properties will influence the bowels and a gentle movement will result. Its stimulating properties will pleasantly relieve the mucous lining of the stomach and bowels of all dryness. A few days will generally be sufficient.

In eruptive diseases such as scarlet fever, measles, etc., use as above, or combine with marigold flowers. At the same time, sponge the body with vinegar and warm water daily.

For worms, take hyssop tea 3 times daily before meals.

In hot infusion, it influences the circulation giving a good outward flow of blood.

To relieve coryza, inhale the steam.

Hyssop can be used either as an infusion or decoction. The infusion made from 1 oz. herb steeped in 1 pt. boiling water is taken frequently in wine-glassful doses.

Although popular medicinally, hyssop has also been used in salads, soups, stews, and in honey. Also used to flavor the liquor, Chartreuse.

During the plagues and pestilences, hyssop was carried in bouquets and strewn about as a prophylactic against infectious diseases.

Hyssop is mentioned often in the Bible. The most interesting are the following: Psalm 51:7—(David sings a prayer for forgiveness and sanctification) "Purge me with hyssop and I shall be clean."

St. John 19:29—(At the Crucifixion, Jesus said, I thirst)—"They filled a sponge with vinegar, and put it upon hyssop, and put it to His mouth."

GROUND IVY (*Glechoma Hederacea*)

Ground ivy is a common wild plant with a strong aromatic odor and a bitter, acrid taste.

From the time of the Anglo-Saxons, ground ivy has figured conspicuously in domestic medicine. The HERB is used.

It is a gently stimulating tonic to the mucous membrane, especially that of the kidneys and of the respiratory tubuli. Also useful in kidney diseases, indigestion, the liver, and in cough and pulmonary troubles generally. The secernents all, more or less, feel its influence. Added to cough syrups it is of much value to persons inclined to be bilious.

A wash made from ground ivy is useful in severe skin eruptions of long standing.

Where expectoration is too free in chronic bronchitis and phthisis, ground ivy will be found useful.

For a tumor, abscesses, gatherings or other sores, use a poultice of the following: 2 oz. ground ivy, 1 oz. each camomile flowers, and fresh yarrow.

An infusion of the leaves is very beneficial in lead colic (poisoning), and painters use it as a preventative.

A hot infusion influences the circulation toward the surface and sustains the nervous system.

The herb infused in wine is considered an old remedy in sciatica.

The infusion is made with 1 oz. herb or leaves steeped in 1 pt. boiling water, taken in wine-glassful doses. Covered till cold, strained and sweetened with honey, it may be taken liberally as a cooling beverage.

JUNIPER (*Juniperis Communis*)

The juniper is a native of Europe but has become naturalized in this country and grows wild in most parts of the U.S.

The FRUITS and TOPS of the juniper are the only official

parts. Although equal to the European in appearance, the best berries are imported from So. Europe. The fruits do not ripen until late in the 2nd year.

They have an agreeable, somewhat aromatic odor and a sweetish, warm, bitter, slightly turpentine taste. They owe their medical virtues chiefly to an essential oil. The berries impart their virtues to water and alcohol. The tops contain similar virtues.

Influencing primarily the kidneys and the bladder, the berries are best suited to torpid conditions of the renal organs. It increases the urine in retention of the urine, and in gravel they are often useful. They may also be used in cases of pain in the lumbar region, catarrh of the bladder, and have some reputation in cases where uric acid is retained in the system, also in sluggish conditions of the uterine function, in typhoid fever, dropsy, cystic catarrh, and renal congestion. They have been recommended in scorbutic and cutaneous diseases, and atonic conditions of the alimentary canal and uterus.

Used in conjunction with other remedies, they have a place in the treatment of rheumatism and sciatica. It is, however, NOT well to use them in acute inflamed conditions unless combined with gravel root in excess.

The oil of juniper, extracted from both the berries and the wood, has long been used as a home remedy for backache and kidney troubles in doses of 4 to 6 drops on a little sugar.

Although more stimulating, the oil very much resembles the berries in properties and may be used for the same general purpose. With vaseline or glycerine, it is useful on irritated surfaces.

In suppression of the menstrual flow from cold and exposure, the cold infusion will be useful: crush 1 oz. berries and infuse in 1 pt. boiling water. Cover until cold. Strain and take wine-glassful doses every 3 or 4 hours.

A very fine diuretic mixture is made as follows: ½ oz. each juniper berries, buchu leaves, white poplar bark, and marshmallow root simmered in 2 pts. water for 15 min. Strain and take 3 or 4 T. 3 or 4 times daily.

When the berries are not available the fluid extract may be used; mix 1 oz. each FE juniper and FE gravel rt. with 2 oz. syrup of ginger and take 1 t. 4 times daily.

They may be taken in substance, triturated with sugar, in the dose of 1 or 2 drachms., repeated 3 or 4 times a day; but the infusion is a more convenient form. It is prepared by crushing 1 oz. bruised berries and steeping in 1 pt. boiling water. Cover till cold. Strain and take in wine-glassful doses every 3 or 4 hrs. Extracts are prepared from the berries and taken in the dose of 1 or 2 Dr., but in consequence of the evaporation of the essential oils, they are probably not stronger than the berries in substance.

Juniper berries form an ingredient in gin and in food seasoning. In the old days, juniper was used as a strewing herb, the pine-like color of which was considered extremely healthy.

Tradition has it that when the Virgin and the infant Christ were fleeing from Herod into Egypt, they took refuge behind a juniper bush.

The wood was formerly used for fumigation.

LADY'S SLIPPER (Cypripedium Pubescens)

Ladies' slipper grows in the rich woods and meadows in the U.S.

The ROOT is the part used in medicine. The odor is lightly valerianic (it is sometimes called American valerian); the taste is sweetish, acrid, bitter, and aromatic.

The root is almost a pure nervine, accounting for the name of "nerve root" also given to it. It spends all of its medicinal properties on the nervous system.

It is almost a pure relaxant and can be used to excellent advantage in the delirium of fevers, either alone or in a combination of 2 parts ladies' slipper and 1 part lobelia, making an infusion and taking a dessert-spoonful occasionally. It relaxes nerve tension and permits a refreshing sleep.

In the delirium of typhoid fever, add a little cayenne. It will relieve brain irritation and refreshing sleep will result.

In nerve irritation, where there is much restlessness and inability to sleep, use ladies' slipper and lobelia in equal parts. In dysmenorrhea and uterine irritation, add some cayenne. Infuse or make into pills with extract of boneset.

In hysteria, it is one of the best remedies. With convulsions, add asafoetida, a little ginger, and a little lobelia.

It is valuable in nervous headache, sleeplessness, or any irritable condition arising from enfeebled nerve conditions. Use ladies' slipper 2 parts and skullcap 1 part in this condition and in a case of irritable nervous depression. If the stomach is involved, use by enema.

Those overworked and worried can secure help by taking small and frequent doses of the simple infusion.

In some cases of insomnia, an injection of ladies' slipper may be given when retiring, and at times a little lobelia may be added. This combination will give good results in nymphomania and assist in preventing emissions.

In parturition, the following will relieve a rigid os uteri and calm nervous irritability: 3 parts ladies' slipper, 2 parts raspberry leaves, 1 part bruised ginger. Infuse 1 oz. in 1 pt. boiling water and take a wine-glassful every hour. If more stimulation is needed, add a little cayenne.

For colic and after-pains, use 3 parts ladies' slipper, 2 parts wild yam, 1 part ginger. Infuse 1 oz. in 1 pt. boiling water and take as required. It will give favorable results. In case of postpartem hemorrhage, however, omit the ginger and add either trillium, cayenne, or black haw.

For rheumatism, combine with some stimulant.

In low states of typhus fever, congestions with nerve irritation, and similar conditions, it is too relaxing to be used alone; combine with an excess of cayenne and golden seal.

A soothing syrup for children and for neuralgia is made as follows: all FE, 2 oz. ladies' slipper, 1 oz. each skullcap, prickly ash, and pleurisy root, 1 oz. tincture lobelia and 1 oz. essence of aniseed. Mix and take from ¼ to 1 t. in warm water, sweetened, or in a little catnip tea.

In the presence of putrescence, ladies' slipper will relieve irritation of the nervous system.

In cranial or abdominal pain, the following is a soothing nervine for child and adult: all FE, ladies' slipper 4 dr., 1 dr. each skullcap, catnip, wild yam and 4 oz. syrup of ginger.

If ladies' slipper is used with tonic medicine, its power is increased.

It is of course understood that if the system is loaded with poisons, causing nerve irritation, measures should be taken to eliminate the offending matter as ladies' slipper will not do this.

LICORICE (Glycyrrhiza Glabra)

Licorice is a native of So. Europe, growing in the U.S. in rich, moist soil.

It is without smell and of a sweet mucilaginous taste which is sometimes mingled with a slight degree of acrimony. Before being used, the ROOT should always be deprived of its outer skin, which is somewhat acrid and without possession of any of the virtues of the root.

Licorice root is an old and exceedingly popular remedy. It is well adapted to catarrhal affections, coughs, sore throat, hoarseness, chest and lung troubles, and is soothing to irritated, mucous membranes of the bowels and urinary passages.

An excellent old family remedy for persistent tickling cough was made as follows: ½ C. linseed (the whole seed) and 1 oz. licorice simmered in 1 qt. water to the consistency of syrup and strained. Children find this pleasant to take and can be given to them in doses up to 1 teacupful; adults can take the decoction freely. Can be taken warm or cold.

Licorice is frequently used as an addition to decoctions to cover an unpleasant taste or bitterness and makes them more acceptable to the stomach. When a compound is made for the lungs of such as boneset, elecampane, wild cherry, and white horehound, adding a little licorice will not only improve the remedy but cover up an unpleasant taste.

Licorice is best taken in the form of a decoction which may be prepared by boiling 1 oz. of the bruised root for a few minutes in 1 pt. water. By long boiling, the acrid principle is extracted.

The powdered root is also used in the preparation of pills, either to give them due consistence, or to cover their surfaces and prevent them from adhering together.

The extract of licorice is made in more than one grade. Always use the best. It is practically all soluble in water.

WHITE POND LILY (Nymphea Odorata)

This plant is common in ponds throughout most of the U.S.

The ROOT is the medicinal part. The taste is mucilaginous and astringent with no odor.

White pond lily tones the mucous membrane throughout, leaving a soothing effect. It removes morbid matter from the system and lessens mucus discharges.

In bowel complaints where an astringent is needed, in diarrhea, dysentery, and cystic catarrh, the decoction is most useful. Also in catarrh of the bladder and irritation of the prostate.

It is one of the best in poultices for inflamed tumors and sores, and is frequently combined in equal parts with crushed linseed or powdered red elm.

For external applications, the decoction can be used as a lotion for sore legs and sores generally.

In infants bowel troubles, thrush, aphthous sore mouth, sore and inflamed gums, and as a gargle in putrid sore throat and throat irritations, it is very healing.

In pharyngitis, used internally, lily and cascara sagrada in equal parts will clean the mucous membrane, heal and soothe the ulcerations and inflammation.

Very useful in local application in leucorrhea, prolapsus uteri, relaxed vagina, ulceration of the cervix, and gleet. Can be used as a vaginal douche.

It forms a good wash for sore eyes, purulent ophthalmia, and scrofulous sores.

The powdered root is soothing dusted on chafed and excoriated surfaces and upon irritable chancres and excoriations of the prepuce and vulva.

A decoction of 1 oz. of root boiled in 1 pt. water for 20 min. is taken internally in wine-glassful doses.

White pond lily is NOT the best remedy to use when there is a tendency to constipation.

LINSEED (*Linum Usitatissimum*)

Originally from Egypt, this plant is now cultivated in the U.S.

The fibre of linseed has been used for centuries in the manufacture of textiles. The roasted seeds are eaten as a food by the Abyssinians, and the cake which remains after the expression of the oil is used as a highly nutritious food for cattle.

Both the SEEDS and the OIL expressed from them are official. They have a mucilaginous taste, slightly unpleasant and without odor.

The mucilage obtained by infusing the entire seeds in boiling water, in the proportion of ½ oz. to 1 pt., is very useful in catarrh, dysentery, nephritic and calculous complaints, stranguary, and other irritated and inflammatory affections, especially of the mucous membrane of the lungs (respiratory tract), intestines (alvine tract), and urinary passages.

For the respiratory tract, it promotes expectoration. For

70

coughs and colds, use the sweetened hot infusion. Take in wine-glassful doses.

For the alvine tract, use it cold. It is soothing, healing, and a tonic in dysentery, diarrhea, and cholera infantum.

The decoction forms a superior laxative enema.

The ground seeds are sold under the name of flaxseed meal.

The meal mixed with hot water forms an excellent poultice. For bronchitis, ulcers, abscesses, and boils, add a little powdered lobelia seed. For general use combine with red elm bark.

The oil meal (what is left after the oil has been pressed out of the ground seed) is frequently used as a poultice. In bronchitis and pneumonia, it is excellent for the lungs. Lobelia, mullein, or cayenne may be added as desired. For boils and abscesses, add red elm bark.

The raw oil is very valuable. Internally it will prove cathartic. Combined with pulverized red elm, it is a most valuable preparation for an external application on burns and scalds. Never allow the surface to become uncovered or dry until thoroughly healed. Wipe off any pus that may accumulate, remove dead flesh, and cover again with the above. Good also on gunpowder burns. Use nervines, if necessary.

An excellent linseed tea is made with 8 oz. each linseed and rock candy, 3 lemons, pared and sliced, added to 2 qts. boiling water. Strain after it has cooled.

The usual infusion is made with 1 t. seed steeped in 1 C. boiling water.

LOBELIA *(Lobelia Inflata)*

Native to the northeastern U.S., lobelia is now growing throughout all the states.

All parts of it are possessed of medicinal activity, but the ROOT and inflated capsules (SEEDS) are the most powerful. The plant should be collected in August and September when the capsules are numerous and should be carefully dried. The herb must be placed upon its end when drying so the seeds do not drop out of the capsules. It may be kept whole or in powder. In the seed is a volatile oil.

The dried lobelia has a slight odor when chewed, though first without much taste, soon produces a burning, acrid impression upon the posterior parts of the tongue and palate, very closely

71

resembling that produced by tobacco and attended, in like manner, with a flow of saliva and a nauseating effect upon the stomach. The powder is of a green color. The PLANT yields its active properties readily to water and alcohol. The seeds must be crushed.

It is also called "Indian tobacco" and "vomit root." As an emetic, it is very powerful.

Lobelia is among the medicines which were much employed by the Indians in this country. It is considered one of the most valuable remedies and is extensively employed. It is claimed there is nothing known to man that will so effectively clear the air passages of the lungs of viscid matter.

The disease in which it has proved most useful is spasmodic asthma, the paroxysms of which it often greatly mitigates and sometimes wholly relieves, even when not given in doses sufficiently large to promote active vomiting.

Lobelia is one of the greatest equalizers of the circulation and gives a full outward flow of blood. Its influence reaches every organ and almost, if not quite, every tissue of the body. In influencing the circulation, it also influences the nerves; sympathetic, central, and spinal. Its range is wide, especially in acute troubles.

Lobelia is best suited when arterial action is strong and when given in more or less putrescent conditions. Its continuance should be brief, only sufficient to cleanse and then use more stimulating treatment. Lobelia is NOT BEST in nervous prostration, paralysis, gangrene, or shock.

Lobelia is a most efficient relaxant, influencing mucus, serous, nervous, and muscular structures. It influences the glandular system, the fauces, and the respiratory tubuli. It is a good rule to always take a stimulant before using lobelia or to combine a stimulant with it.

It is used in cough, bronchitis, asthma, whooping cough, pneumonia, hysteria, convulsions, suspended animation, tetanus, febrile troubles, spasmodic or membranous croup, pleuritis, hepatitis, peritonitis, nephritis, phrenitis, otitis, ophthalmia, rheumatism, occlusion of the gall ducts, strangulated hernia, rigid os uteri, and is extremely useful as an emetic when the stomach should be thoroughly cleaned.

In puerperal convulsions, use the following: 2 dr. FX. lobelia,

4 Dr. Fl. X ladies' slipper, ½ Dr. tincture cayenne, and simple syrup sufficient to make 6 oz. Dose—1 t. every ½ hour.

It is one of the best aids in surgery where relaxation is required, especially in dislocations for which take regularly and frequently and apply locally.

In cases of infantile coughs and bronchitis, when the child seems likely to be suffocated by phlegm, a dose will remove the obstruction.

In convulsions, combine with blue cohosh.

The acid tincture of lobelia is made as follows: lobelia herb and crushed seed each 2 oz. and 1 pt. best malt vinegar. Steep in a closely stoppered bottle for 10 days to 2 weeks, shaking every day. Strain and bottle for use. If the vinegar is brought to the boiling point before adding, it will be ready to use at once.

This also has been used as an external application, rubbing it between the shoulders and on the chest in asthma and most helpful in cases where breathing has been most difficult.

To make a pleasant, yet efficient remedy for croup, whooping cough, and asthma, fill a bottle ¾ full of the acid tincture and add sugar or honey to fill the bottle. Shake until dissolved.

The acid tincture can be added to horehound, hyssop, sage, or other teas (1 t. to 1 C.) in coughs, asthma, and colds. Can be used as an emetic if the stomach should be cleaned.

What is known as anti-spasmodic tincture is used in many violent cases such as epilepsy, convulsions, lockjaw, delirium tremens, fainting, hysteria, cramps, suspended animation, spasms, and is considered unequalled in the whole realm of therapeutic remedies in these cases.

It is valuable in sluggish cases as it arouses the system to dislodge semi-putrescent material and to quickly stimulate and equalize the circulation. It is excellent in sick-headache, dyspepsia, and in the incipiency of apoplexy. When life hangs in the balance or where effects are required on short notice, the anti-spasmodic tincture can be relied on.

The anti-spasmodic tincture is made as follows: all in powder—1 oz. each crushed lobelia seed and herb, skunk cabbage root, skullcap, gum myrrh, valerian, and ½ oz. cayenne. Infuse for 1 week in 1 qt. best brandy in closely corked, wide-necked bottle. Shake well daily. After 1 week, strain and press out the clear liquid, it is then ready for use.

A drop or two on the tip of the finger, thrusting the finger into the mouth of a baby in convulsions, has stopped them at once.

Dominion Herbal College writes in their Post Graduate Course as follows: "In mucous and spasmodic croup, the anti-spasmodic tincture must be administered promptly and in full teaspoonful doses in warm water and repeated every 10 to 15 minutes until free vomiting ensues.

"Where the case is severe or the anti-spasmodic tincture is difficult to administer, as in the case of infants, rub well into the neck, chest, and between the shoulders. At the same time 2 or 3 drops of the tincture in a raw state should be placed in the mouth and washed down with 1 t. dose of warm water and the patient kept warm in bed. Repeat every 1 or 2 hours, if necessary.

"In scarlet fever and other febrile conditions, in typhoid, typhus, spotted (spinal meningitis), black or slow fever, especially malignant scarlet fever use 1 t. anti-spasmodic tincture in a little warm water and give every ½ hr. until the patient is easier. Then get 2 qts. hot water and 1 qt. best malt vinegar. Mix and wash entire body, then wipe dry. Be sure patient is kept warm. Then give 1 t. of anti-spasmodic tincture in warm herb tea every 2 hrs. Wash with vinegar and warm water every day." He claims scores of scarlet fever patients were saved with this method after hope was given up for their recovery.

"In rheumatic fever, rub the whole body from neck to toes with the anti-spasmodic tincture, and if the case is bad, so that he cannot sit up or move arms or legs, give 1 t. anti-spasmodic tincture in a little hot water every ½ hr. until free perspiration ensues. Keep patient in bed, allow to cool down, and then wash the whole body down with vinegar and hot water. After this give anti-spasmodic tincture in teaspoonful doses in hot water every 2 hrs. for 1 day, then every 3 hrs. for a few days. Sponge down daily with hot water and vinegar."

For rattlesnake bite take equal parts of anti-spasmodic tincture and tincture lobelia, FE skullcap and FE valerian, ¼ t. in warm water every 5 min., in a strong infusion of black cohosh.

A very useful preparation is the syrup of lobelia: boil 2½ oz. lobelia herb in 2 pints water down to 1 pt. Strain and dissolve in the liquid by low heat 2# sugar. This is useful in coughs, etc. but will be emetic if taken in large doses.

The acid syrup of lobelia is made as follows: 1 pint each lobelia syrup and malt vinegar mixed together. Dose ¼ t. is excellent for asthmatic cough.

Lobelia capsules are made as follows: all in powder, 1 oz. each lobelia seed, lobelia herb, cayenne, aniseed, and 2 oz. gum arabic. Mix and fill into #4 capsules.

These are useful in dyspepsia, rheumatism, inflammation, asthma, consumption, chills, jaundice, and fevers. Dose, 4 to 10 a day as required.

In scarlet fever, etc., when necessary, dissolve a quantity of the contents of a dozen of the capsules in ¾ C. hot water and give as the anti-spasmodic tincture, following directions about bathing the body.

Where lobelia is used as an emetic, always have some stimulating tea before. Peppermint or composition tea is useful in this connection.

Very weak persons can take emetics when they are needed; even an occasional emetic may be given to consumptives. Also valuable in puerperal fevers. Give to cleanse and stop; repeat only as required.

The oil is less stimulating and less likely to produce emesis.

For hysterical coughs use oil of lobelia and oil of ginger each 3 drops, blue cohosh and black cohosh each 1½ grs. Triturate on sugar, take 3 doses, 15 min. apart.

To make lobelia pills, mix together the following all powdered, 1½ gr. lobelia seed, 1 gr. ladies' slipper, ½ gr. cayenne with extract of boneset of sufficient quantity to make pills. Dose, 1 pill every 4 hrs. as required. This is considered an excellent preparation where profound relaxation is desired without emesis. It is excellent in peritonitis, lung, and bronchial troubles, especially for bronchial cough and painful conditions in any part of the body.

A paste is made of lobelia and bi-carbonate of soda rubbed well into inflamed or poisoned sores. Keep surface moistened with lobelia tincture. The pain will cease quickly.

In a case of strangulated hernia, a strong decoction was administered by the rectum, as a substitute for a narcotic.

Lobelia may be used in substance, i.e., the powdered herb or seed, in Fl X, acid tincture, infusion, decoction, pills, or capsules, in syrup, by enema, and in poultice.

The dose of the powder is 3–10 grs. and as an emetic is from 5 to 20 gr. to be repeated, if necessary. The tincture is most frequently used, and this is considered as the U.S. official preparation. The full dose of this preparation for an adult is ½ fl. oz. though in asthmatic cases it is better administered in the quantity of 1–2 fl. dr., repeated every 2 or 3 hrs. till its effects are experienced.

The infusion is made of 1 oz. powdered herb in 1 pt. boiling water. Allow to stand covered. Take in doses of ½ to 1 wineglassful.

All accumulations of mucous are instantly removed after a full dose of the infusion and many lives have been saved by its timely use.

Dominion College states: "We believe that lobelia is one of the finest remedies with which a kind Providence has blessed mankind."

PURPLE LOOSESTRIFE (*Lythrum Salicaria*)

Purple loosestrife was introduced into the U.S. from Europe.

The WHOLE PLANT is medicinal, and is dried for use. In this state, it is inodorous and has an herbaceous, somewhat astringent taste. It renders boiling water very mucilaginous.

Purple loosestrife, although an astringent, does not leave the tissues dry, but promotes the secretion of the mucous membrane, leaving them moist. This renders it valuable in hepatic troubles, typhoid, constipation, and tends to strengthen the muscular tissues.

Its influence extends to the mucous, secretory, vascular, and nervous systems. Also the liver, kidneys, bladder, and the biliary duct.

It is used in fevers, dysentery, cholera infantum, cholera morbus, hemorrhages, leucorrhea, sores, and ulcers. The herb is considered superior to eyebright in preserving sight and restoring clouded vision, hurts and blows on the eyes, providing the crystalline humour is not injured or destroyed. Distilled water is used.

76

Combined with white pond lily, bayberry bark, water agrimony (bur marigold) and a little ginger, it is very good in leucorrhea and passive bleeding of all kinds.

It was widely used in England in the cholera epidemics of 1848, 1852-3, 1864, and 1868. It is claimed to be of benefit no matter if in the 1st, 2nd, 3rd or 4th stages or even the very last stages of this disease. From the moment it enters the stomach, the irritation seems to be allayed, hepatic and biliary derangements corrected, and the mucous secretions restored to their normal conditions; the kidney and bladder are strengthened, nervous excitement is abated, diaphoresis is promoted, and the skin, instead of being dry and clammy, becomes soft and moist. It also allays the spasmodic cramps, and the patient is eventually brought to rest and sleep.

The method used in cholera and fever cases is as follows: boil 3 oz. purple loosestrife (fresh herb) or 1½ oz. dried herb and 1 oz. crushed ginger in 3 pts. water to 1¾ pts., strain and take a small cupful every ½ hr. until the patient feels easier, then take just warm as the case indicates.

In quinsy and sore throat, use a warm gargle of the decoction. Taken internally at the same time would be beneficial.

Purple loosestrife has long been popular in Ireland and Sweden in diarrhea and chronic dysentery.

Also excellent as an ointment for sores.

The usual decoction of the root is made by boiling 1 oz. in 1 pt. water, taken in a dose of 2 fl. oz. The dose of the powdered herb is about 1 dr. taken 2 or 3 times daily.

AMERICAN MANDRAKE *(Podophyllum Peltatum)*

Indigenous, this plant grows luxuriantly in moist shady woods and in low marshy grounds. It is the only species belonging to the genus.

The leaves are said to be poisonous.

The fruit has a subacid, sweetish, peculiar taste, agreeable to some palates and may be eaten freely. From its color and shape, it is sometimes called WILD LEMON. The Indians were well acquainted with the virtues of this plant.

The ROOT is the official portion and is said to be most efficient when collected after the falling of the leaves. It shrinks considerably in drying. It is nearly inodorous, but in powder form it has a sweetish, not unpleasant smell. The taste is at first sweetish, afterwards bitter, nauseating, and slightly acrid. The decoction and tincture are bitter. In its fresh state it is an acrid, nauseating, and altogether drastic agent. When dry, this objectionable feature is, to a very great extent, dissipated. It is a powerful article and should not be used in too large or too frequent doses or it will gripe and cause distress, watery evacuations, and uneasiness in the pelvis and bowels.

American mandrake is an active and certain cathartic producing copious liquid discharges without much griping or other unpleasant effect. It is decidedly a cholagogue and a cathartic in from 6 to 10 hrs. If used as a cathartic, add a little ginger but use no sugar.

Its influence is particularly noted on the salivary glands, mucous membrane if not irritated, gall ducts, liver, and kidneys. Because of its influence on the pelvic organs, it is UNFIT to use in the pregnant state.

It is highly valuable in all chronic, scrofulous and dyspeptic complaints, dropsy, bilious and liver disorders. In congestions of the liver, about 10 gr. powdered mandrake and 5 gr. powdered cloves are taken in honey. The Fl. X may be taken in doses of 5 to 30 drops.

The resinoid, podophyllin, is much used now. It is valuable in liquifying the gall in the relief of gall stones for which purpose it is best taken in syrup of ginger or in capsules. Take large doses every few minutes. It will not nauseate nor produce catharsis until the parts are eased and the gall liquified. Occasional doses must be taken to maintain a liquid condition. In small doses it is useful in jaundice. It acts upon the liver in the same manner as mercury, but is superior to it.

The preparation of the root is to be preferred to those of the resin, podophyllin.

In minute doses, frequently repeated, podophyllum (Fl X) is said to diminish the frequency of the pulse, to relieve cough, and for these effects is sometimes used in spitting up of blood, catarrh, and other pulmonary affections.

The doses of the powdered root is 2–10 grs.

The simple infusion is made of 1 t. root, cut small, to 1 pt. boiling water. Take 1 t. at a time, as required.

Note: American mandrake must not be confused with the English mandrake which is called white bryony *(Bryonia Alba)*.

MARSHMALLOW *(Althea Officinalis)*

This plant is found in moist places in the U.S. In Europe it is largely cultivated for medicinal use.

The whole plant abounds in mucilage, which is especially abundant in the root. The root has a feeble odor and a mild mucilaginous taste. It yields its mucilage to water by decoction. It should be kept dry or it will give a yellowish decoction of unpleasant odor.

The virtues of marshmallow are exclusively those of a demulcent. The ROOTS and the LEAVES have the same properties, but the roots are the stronger.

A decoction of the root is very soothing in irritations and inflammations of the mucous membranes and in coughs due to colds, pharyngitis, laryngitis, and acute and chronic pulmonary troubles. Also in dysentery, diarrhea, typhoid fever, gonorrhea, stranguary, vaginal douche, cystitis, urethritis, and nephritis. In irritations of the kidneys and urinary tract, its soothing effect helps to bring away stone and gravel.

It is most effective in hemorrhage from the urinary organs. For this boil the powdered root in milk and drink freely.

In obstinate inflammation, where mortification threatens, make a poultice of the boiled crushed or powdered root and apply as hot as can be borne. The efficacy of this poultice is such that the root is also called mortification root. The addition of red elm is an advantage.

The leaves and the roots, bruised and boiled, are quite commonly used in external applications as a fomentation or poultice in all manner of swellings, pain, inflammation, abscesses, and festering sores. Make a strong decoction with leaves or roots and wring out a flannel and apply as hot as can be borne for one hour at a time. Repeat as frequently as needed.

For gathered breasts, gum boils, and neuralgia add chamomile flowers and poppy heads.

For sprains and swellings, add ragwort.

A good covering for burns, scalds, and denuded surfaces with the addition of raw linseed oil.

As a wash and poultice in ophthalmia, add lobelia.

As a wash in inflammation of the eyes, the following is recommended: boil 1 oz. marshmallow root and ¼ oz. red raspberry leaves in 1½ pts. water down to 1 pt. Strain and bathe the eyes with the decoction cold ½ doz. times daily.

The powdered root is considered excellent for enriching milk in nursing mothers, as well as increasing the flow. Boil the powdered root in milk and drink freely.

The usual infusion is made of 1 oz. leaves in 1 pt. boiling water, taken frequently in wine-glassful doses.

The syrup of marshmallow is made by boiling 8 oz. fresh root, sliced, in 4 pints water. Strain and add 2½# sugar. Dose ½ oz. to 1 oz. The lozenges are also useful in hoarseness, coughs, etc. They are made by adding a little more sugar and mucilage of gum tragacanth to the syrup.

ICELAND MOSS (Cetraria Islandica)

A native of Britain, this plant is found in the mountains and the sandy plains of New England. It received its name from the abundance in which it prevails in Iceland. It is a parasite like the mistletoe.

It is inodorous, has a mucilaginous bitter taste and, when wet, smells like seaweed.

Macerated in water, it absorbs more than its own weight and, if the water is warm, renders it bitter. Boiling water extracts the soluble principle which gelatinizes on cooling.

The Icelanders and Laplanders use it as a food. The gum and starch contained in the moss render it very nutritious. They powder it and make it into bread or boil it with milk. It is first macerated in water to release the bitter principle. This procedure is not recommended, if used as a medicine.

In addition to being an excellent diet for a patient, it is a very useful medicine.

Because of its demulcent, nutritious, and tonic properties, Iceland moss is particularly applicable to affections of the mucous membrane of the lungs and bowels, especially in debilitated conditions of the digestive system, in dyspepsia, to improve the appetite and digestion, and of the system generally.

It is most extensively used in pulmonary consumption and in all pulmonary complaints such as coughs, expectoration of blood, chronic bronchitis, chronic catarrh, chronic dysentery and diarrhea, leucorrhea and other debilitating troubles attended with copious and debilitating expectoration and especially when the discharges are of a purulent character. This includes external ulcers and debility following an acute disease.

Iceland moss acquired a reputation in pulmonary consumption and in the coughing up and spitting up of blood and bloody mucus. It was extensively used in these conditions. Modern pathology deems other herbs more suitable to tuberculosis.

Iceland moss is usually employed in the form of a decoction of 1 oz. boiled in 1½ pts. water, strained while hot. It thickens upon cooling and acquires a gelatinous consistence.

Its soothing influence, coupled with its strengthening properties, renders it a suitable drink both as a medicine and as a diet. It can be taken as a gruel or in smaller doses as medicine. Milk may be added as a diet drink. The powder is sometimes used in dose of 30 gr. to 1 dr. An addition of chocolate will make it an excellent beverage with meals.

IRISH MOSS (Chondrus Crispus)

Irish moss grows on submerged rocks, therefore, it is actually not a moss but a seaweed. It is found quite commonly on the shores of Europe and the U.S.

The taste is mucilaginous and saline; the odor is that of a seaweed. It is bleached by exposure to the sun and repeated washings.

Its properties are similar to Iceland moss. It is used principally in chronic coughs and bronchitis, pneumonia, and consumption. It is very useful and perfectly safe in consumption of the bowels. Also in irritating diseases of the bladder and kidneys.

A diet drink is made by boiling 1 oz. in 1½ pts. milk. Strain, sweeten to taste, and add a dash of cinnamon or nutmeg, if desired.

Medicinal dose—1 t. dried PLANT to 1 C. boiling water.

Inferior grades are fed to cattle.

MOTHERWORT (Leonurus Cardiaca)

In Japan, this plant is called "herb of life."

A member of the mint family and originating in Europe and Asia, motherwort has become naturalized in the U.S.

It has a peculiar aromatic, not disagreeable, odor and a

slightly aromatic bitter taste. It yields its properties to water and alcohol.

Motherwort is a very useful PLANT and a pleasant and a very excellent tonic. In cases where the lumbar region and the pelvis are troubled in tardy menstruation, it will tone the generative organs and quiet nervous irritability, gently promoting the menstrual flow and toning the uterine membrane. It should be given in warm infusion.

A hot infusion promotes a good outward circulation. It is useful in amenorrhea and in dysmenorrhea when congestion is present and in hysteria and palpitation when more or less chlorotic.

For the chlorotic, who have some scrofulous or other impurity of the blood current, the following will be useful—all Fl X —motherwort and burdock seeds ½ Dr. each, prickly ash ½ Dr., yellow parilla 2 Dr. in 4 oz. simple syrup.

Motherwort is NOT the proper remedy for the pregnant nor for those given to too free menstruation. It is useful in cases of after-pain when the lochia is quite scanty.

A cold infusion is a gentle heart tonic in heart diseases or weakness and in recovery from fevers. In delirium and nervous excitement attendant upon fevers, it will quiet the nerves and promote a restful sleep.

Its tonic properties are serviceable in gastric and intestinal indigestion; improving the appetite and assisting digestion.

In these conditions, the following is often effective: motherwort and dandelion Rt. 1 oz. ea., golden seal Rt. and centaury ½ oz. ea., ginger Rt. ¼ oz. Simmer in 3 pts. water down to 1 qt. Strain and take 3 T. 3 or 4 times daily.

In simple vaginitis, motherwort has been used as a vaginal douche.

The infusion is made by steeping 1 oz. herb in 1 pt. water and taken in wine-glassful doses.

MULLEIN (*Verbascum Thapsus*)

Mullein was known as the torch flower in the days of the Romans because the soldiers dipped the plant into tallow to make torches.

Mullein is common throughout the U.S. It is a naturalized plant, introduced originally from Europe.

The LEAVES and FLOWERS are used but the leaves are preferred. Both have a slight, somewhat narcotic smell, which, in the dried flowers, becomes agreeable. Their taste is mucilaginous, herbaceous, slightly bitter, but very feeble. They impart their medicinal virtues to water by infusion.

Where the effusions and accumulations are desired to be absorbed and carried off, mullein is remarkable in its influence on the absorbents.

The leaves and the flowers are very useful in pulmonary diseases, coughs, consumption, hemorrhage of the lungs, in dysentery, and in diarrhea, the demulcent properties strengthening the bowels. The ordinary infusion may be used. In diarrhea, however, if there is bleeding from the bowels, boil 1 oz. of mullein in 1 pt. milk, sweeten, if desired. Strain and take in ½ teacupful doses after each stool.

Mullein is one of the most valuable herbs in its influence upon the glandular system, the serous and the mucus structures. It is especially valuable in glandular swellings, hepatization or thickening of lung tissues, phthisis, asthma, hayfever, catarrhal coughs, coughs due to colds, pleuritic effusions, mild catarrhs, pleuritis, cellular and synovial dropsy, scrofulous and other swellings, chronic abscesses, and all forms of dropsies.

In mumps and some severe and vicious glandular swellings, a fomentation of leaves has been most successfully used.

In bronchitis or croupy cough, apply the following over the lungs; 2 oz. Mullein, ¼ oz. lobelia, 1 t. cayenne, simmered in 2 qts. water 15 min. Foment as warm as convenient and take the following: all FE, mullein, poke, elder flowers, life everlasting each 2 Dr. in 4 oz. simple syrup.

The leaves are also employed externally, steeped in hot water in the treatment of sprains, bruises, soreness of the chest, and painful chronic abscesses.

In a case of painful and swollen joints, cover a quantity of mullein (either green or dried) with boiling vinegar. Cover and simmer slowly for 20 to 30 min. Strain and add a little tincture cayenne and FE lobelia. Foment and it will ease the pains and, in almost every case, reduce the swelling.

For stiff joints and rheumatism, foment with 4 oz. mullein, ½ oz. lobelia herb, ¼ oz. cayenne, 2 qts. vinegar. Bring to a boil and simmer slowly 20 to 30 min.

For external irritations and itching piles, apply a fomentation of the leaves in hot vinegar and water.

In ophthalmia, cover the eyes with a soft cloth wet with ½ oz. mullein, 20 gr. golden seal, 1 dr. lobelia herb, and 6 oz. water.

For nasal congestion and catarrh or throat irritation, place a handful of leaves in an old teapot and cover with hot water. Inhale the steam through the spout.

For inflamed peritonium apply 3 oz. FE mullein and 1 oz. tincture cayenne.

For periostitis, apply 2 Dr. each FE mullein, oil sassafras, oil peppermint, tincture ginger, tincture lobelia, and 4 oz. alcohol.

For dropsied limbs, apply 4 oz. FE mullein, 2½ oz. tincture cayenne, 1 oz. tincture lobelia, and ½ Dr. oil origanum.

For dysentery use 2 Dr. FE mullein, 3 Dr. each FE catnip, and FE ladies' slipper in ½ teacupful tepid water for enema after each stool.

In Europe, an infusion of the flowers, strained to remove the rough hairs, is considerably used in mild catarrhs.

A simple infusion is made of both leaves and flowers, 1 t. to 1 C. boiling water, taken in 1 or 2 C daily doses.

CAUTION: While Mullein has a very powerful influence on the absorbents and is extremely valuable in mumps, glandular swellings, dropsies, etc., it must NOT BE USED IN CANCERS or any other swellings where it would be injurious to have a deposit absorbed.

WHITE OAK (*Quercus Alba*)

The white oak is one of the most magnificent and noble hardwood trees growing in most of the U.S. It is the oak most highly valued for its timber with the exception of the live oak.

The white oak is the one chiefly used in medicine, and the inner portion of the BARK is the official portion. It is not easily pulverized. It has a feeble odor and a rough astringent and bitterish taste. Water and alcohol extracts its active properties.

It is a powerful astringent in internal and external hemorrhage.

Useful in debility, scrofula, intermittent fevers, obstinate chronic diarrhea, and cholera infantum. A decoction can be advantageously employed as a bath when a combined tonic and astringent is desired and the stomach is not disposed to receive medicine kindly, particularly for children.

As an injection or wash in leucorrhea, diarrhea, dysentery, prolapsus uteri, relaxed vagina, by rectum in prolapsus ani, fissures and hemorrhoids, and as a gargle in slight inflammation of the fauces attended with prolapsed uvula, the decoction is often highly useful. Also as a gargle in ulcerated and inflamed throat and in suspicion of a light attack of diphtheria, add a little cayenne or composition powder. It may be taken in decoction internally in small and frequent doses. In acute and chronic diarrhea, add ginger, prickly ash or cayenne, when taken internally.

Reduced to powder and made into a poultice, it is recommended in cases of external gangrene and mortification.

The decoction makes a good wash for sweaty and tender feet, ulcers, sores, bruises, tetters, ringworm, and scaly eruptions, and to prevent the falling out of hair.

It is useful to harden gums prior to fitting with false teeth and is a good wash for sore mouth, spongy and bleeding gums.

A help in goitre would be a towel wrung out of a hot decoction and bound over this swollen gland. Repeat as required.

In tetter on both hands with fissures and bleeding with great swelling and pain use a strong decoction of oak bark. Relief should be had in a few hours.

The bark may be taken internally in the form of a powder, X, or decoction. The dose of the powder is from 30 gr. to 1 Dr., of the X about half as much. The decoction is made of 1 oz. bark in 1 qt. water, boiled down to 1 pt. and taken in wine-glassful doses.

The ACORNS are considered an old remedy for diarrhea. They are grated or powdered and washed down with water. Roasted and ground, acorns have been used as a coffee substitute. They were the staple food for humans in Northern Europe until the popularity of using cereal grains.

Isaiah (BC 740–742)—6:13–"Shall be eaten, as an oak, whose substance is in them, when they cast their leaves; so the holy seed (acorn) shall be the substance thereof."

YELLOW PARILLA (*Menispermum Canadense*)

Also called American sarsaparilla and moonseed, so called from the crescent-shaped seeds.

Yellow parilla grows in most of the Eastern U.S. The taste is bitter and nearly inodorous. It yields its virtues to water and alcohol.

Its influence will be manifest through the mucous membrane, stomach, gall ducts, liver, and small intestines. It has a distinct alterative and tonic influence upon all the secreting organs and will slightly increase the general circulation.

Considered superior to Jamaica sarsaparilla by some as an alterative, it is often used as a substitute in the treatment of scrofula, syphilis, blood diseases, skin troubles, and cutaneous diseases generally.

Yellow parilla is useful in biliousness, atonic indigestion, atonic dyspepsia, glandular swellings, rheumatism, scrofulous and mercurial rheumatism, debility, secondary syphilis, and indolent ulcers. May be combined with yellow dock, burdock root, white oak, dandelion, false bittersweet and poke for added value.

Combined with remedies that have an especial influence upon the respiratory passages, it is very valuable for the lungs, chronic bronchitis, phthisis, and scrofulous conditions, especially in tuberculosis of the lungs, as it will increase expectoration.

As a hepatic alterant, use, all FE., yellow parilla, burdock Rt. and dandelion in equal parts. As an alterative in skin diseases use, all FE, yellow parilla 3 Dr., white ash 4 Dr., false bittersweet 3 Dr., in 4 oz. of syrup of ginger.

The infusion is made of 1 t. ROOT cut small to 1 C. boiling water, drinking 1 C. cold during the day. The Fl. X is believed to more fully represent the healing virtues of the plant.

GARDEN PARSLEY *(Apium Petroselinium)*

The plant is a native of Sardinia and other parts of South Europe, but is now cultivated everywhere in our gardens. It is an old time remedy, much ignored because of its being so common. Truly a very valuable food and not merely a decoration, as it is so often used.

All parts of it contain an essential oil, to which it owes its medicinal virtues, as well as its use in seasoning. The ROOT is the part most used by the pharmacopias, though the SEEDS are at least equally efficient.

It has a pleasant smell and a sweetish slightly aromatic taste, but loses this property by long boiling and by long keeping. For best results it should be used fresh.

The seeds, herb, and root increase the flow when the urine is scanty and are useful in dropsy, (care must be taken in this disease not to push the kidneys to the point of exhaustion) very useful in gravel, the aching back in the lumbar region, stone and congestion of the kidneys. Because the seeds contain apiol, it has been considered safe and efficient in obstructed menstruation and in both ammenorrhea and dysmenorrhea for many generations.

Parsley is a Greek word meaning "stone breaker."

It is very useful in jaundice.

The seeds are sometimes used as carminatives.

The Romans and the Greeks crowned their heroes with garlands of parsley. Also decked their banquet tables with sumptuous parsley garlands to absorb the fumes of too much imbibing. The Greeks considered parsley a sacred herb and made funeral wreaths and planted it profusely over the mounds of newly dug graves so that it might become a green velvety carpet.

Parsley is used freely for culinary purposes and is useful in removing traces of onions and garlic from the breath.

It is also used in coloring some wines and sage cheese.

A French chemist claims the apiol obtained from the seeds proved to be a good substitute for quinine and ergot.

This herb is a source of calcium, thiamin (Vit B-1), riboflavin (Vit B-2), Niacin, and Vit C.

Parsley is very rich in Vit A and in Vit C (3 times as much as an orange) and tremendously high in iron content.

Because of this plentiful supply of vitamins in parsley, it is considered excellent for arthritis pains—the following has been said to be successful: pour 1 qt. boiling water over 1 C. firmly packed parsley, both leaves and stems. Allow to steep 15 min. Strain through a coarse sieve and bottle at once. Cool quickly, keep under refrigeration. Drink a wine-glassful daily in 1 dose or several, undiluted or with water, it does not matter. A dash of salt makes it more palatable.

The usual form of administration is that of a strong infusion. The roots, seeds, or leaves may be used. Can be used either in infusion, decoction, or Fl. X.

EUROPEAN PENNYROYAL *(Mentha Pulegium)*

European pennyroyal belongs to the mint family. It is a native of Europe but is now a common garden plant in the U.S.

The HERB is used. The taste and the odor is like mint.

Its warming influence upon the stomach is very agreeable and sustaining to the capillary circulation.

The infusion will give good results in gas, spasms, colic pains, restless sleep, nervous and cross conditions in feverish children. It will allay nausea and is very useful in menorrhagia.

The hot infusion is a very fine remedy for breaking up colds and feverish conditions. It is considered almost a specific in suppressed or obstructed menstruation, especially when caused by chill or cold.

The hot infusion may be taken freely in eruptive diseases when the eruption is slow in making its appearance. May also be useful as a nervine in spasms, flatulence, hysteria, nausea, and dysmenorrhea in nervous women.

Pennyroyal is considered a specific for sun strokes and for exhaustion from overheating. Give no water to drink and place no ice on the head.

A hot fomentation will be useful for sprains and rheumatism.

The dried leaves can be used as a food flavoring the same as mint.

The oil of pennyroyal is considered a preventative against mosquito and gnat bites. To chase fleas or mosquitoes, strip leaves, put into bags, and sew up. Sprinkle with oil or essence of pennyroyal. Place where needed.

The warm infusion, 1 oz. herb to 1 pt. boiling water, may be taken freely in doses from wine-glassful to ½ teacupful and repeated every one or 2 hours as needed. When the herb cannot be obtained, the OIL of pennyroyal may be given in from 1 to 3 drops in a little warm water or triturated on sugar.

Pennyroyal, the same as other mints, should never be boiled because of its rich volatile oil. Always cover closely to prevent escape of the steam.

The American or mock pennyroyal is *Hedeoma Pulegioides*. The medicinal properties are similar to the European pennyroyal.

PEPPERMINT *(Mentha Piperita)*

A native of Great Britain, peppermint is grown over most of the U.S. Commercially, it is grown in large acreages for the oil which is extracted and used in medicines, perfumes, confections, cold drinks, sauces, and flavoring in many foods of which lamb sauce and jelly is probably the most popular. Benedictine and Creme de Menthe are probably the most popular after-dinner cordials.

There are two varieties of peppermint: The black and the white. It is claimed that the white produces the best oil.

We occasionally find peppermint growing wild. However, in order to maintain its best flavor, the plants should be transplanted every 3 or 4 years. For medical purposes, cut in dry weather just after the flowers appear.

The HERB, both fresh and dried, has a penetrating odor, somewhat resembling camphor. The taste is aromatic, warm, pungent, camphorous, bitterish, and attended with a sensation of coolness when air is admitted into the mouth. These properties depend on a volatile oil which abounds in the herb. Its virtues are imparted to water and more readily to alcohol.

It is soothing to the stomach, allays nausea, relieves spasmodic pains of the stomach and bowels, expels flatus, and is used to cover the taste or qualify the nauseating or griping effects of other medicines. It is useful in colic, dizziness, colds, fever, measles, convulsions, and similar infantile troubles and is especially useful in the cholera of children.

In menstrual obstruction, when hysterical and highly nervous, combine with wood betony in equal parts. Make an infusion and take warm, about a wine glassful every 3 hours.

The following is considered the most reliable treatment of "flu," la grippe, and fevers of inflammations. Pour 1½ pints of boiling water on 1 oz. each peppermint leaves and elder flowers. Cover and keep warm 15 min. Strain, keep covered, and take ½ to 1 C. every 30 to 45 min. until perspiration starts. Then take 2 T. every hour or 2. The important thing is to take it warm and to continue until you perspire freely. You have then broken down congestions and equalized the circulation and you have assisted nature to restore an equilibrium. Stay in bed overnight and in the morning have someone, if possible, sponge the whole body down with equal parts of cider vinegar and warm water. Sponge carefully so as not to catch cold; do one part of the body at a time, keeping the rest of the body covered. This will act as a skin tonic and remove any waste matter.

This can be safely given to children, using smaller dosage and sweetened with honey or a little sugar.

A few fresh leaves placed on the forehead sometimes helps to alleviate a nervous headache and neuralgia and chewing a few leaves often relieves a sick feeling in the stomach.

The writer makes an excellent sauce from fresh mint leaves: chop very fine, pour over them ¼ C. boiling water, add 2 T. sugar, cover closely, and let stand in a cool place ½ hr.; then add juice of 1 lemon or 4 T. cider vinegar, ¾ t. salt. Serve with roast lamb. Best made a day ahead. Strain and reheat.

The OIL is more positive, stimulating and warming but is less relaxing and diffusive than the herb.

The oil of peppermint rubbed upon the surface (skin) will quickly relieve the burning pain of shingles.

An application of the essence of peppermint will relieve pruritis.

The essence of oil of peppermint if taken in small doses, will increase the appetite and prevent fermentation.

Peppermint is a wholesome and refreshing tea for young and old and has been enjoyed for generations. It is still a very popular dinner tea in Germany at the present time.

The fresh herb, bruised and applied over the stomach, often allays sick stomach and is especially useful in the cholera of children.

Peppermint may be given in infusion, but the volatile oil alone, or in some state of preparation, is almost always preferred.

NEVER boil peppermint and always keep the infusion covered, as it is very volatile. Luke 11:42 and also Matt 23:23 (A.D. 33)—Mention is made of mint as a tithe. Evidently this herb was considered valuable in those days.

PIPSISSIWA (Chimaphila Umbellata)

Also called rheumatic weed and false wintergreen.

Pipsissiwa is a native of the U.S. and is found in all the states. It is claimed the name is derived from 2 Greek words—"winter" and "friend." It is official in the U.S.

All parts of the PLANT are endowed with active properties; but the leaves are usually preferred. When fresh and bruised, they exhale a peculiar, rather fragrant odor. When dried they have no odor.

The taste of the leaves is pleasantly bitter, astringent, and sweetish; that of the stems and roots also has a considerable degree of pungency. Boiling water or alcohol extracts their virtues.

It was employed by the Indians in various complaints. From their hands, it passed into those of the European settlers.

It is highly recommended as a remedy in dropsy and is very useful in assisting in cleansing the system, relieving the skin, kidneys, and liver. It is a highly esteemed remedy in scrofula and scurvy both before and after the occurrence of ulceration and in obstinate ill-conditioned ulcers and cutaneous eruptions, especially when connected with a strumous diathesis (tendency to scrofulous tumor). In these cases, Pipsissiwa may be freely used both internally or as a wash. The decoction is preferred. It is made by boiling 2 oz. fresh bruised leaves with 3 pts. water down to 1 qt. and taken 1 pt. in 24 hrs. It is especially valuable in scrofulous debility.

It tones the kidneys in dropsy and will increase the flow of urine. Also useful in cystic catarrh, bladder weakness, calculous and nephritic affections, urinary obstructions, and in general complaints of the urinary passages.

It is particularly useful in cases attended with disordered digestion and general debility in which its tonic property and general acceptability to the stomach prove highly useful auxiliaries to its diuretic powers.

Its influence spreads through the glandular system, the lymphatics, and the secreting organs.

It has been very beneficially used in tumors and phthisis, clearing the blood current from impurities and waste matter. Take in large quantities, if needed.

It has been effectively used in rheumatism and gonorrhea, especially if the trouble be largely from impurities in the blood, cleansing the blood current, and soothing the mucous membrane.

It is valuable not only in its alterative influence, but for its diuretic action in cleansing the mucous membrane of accumulated solids or mucus.

It is useful in syphilis, vaginal and uterine weakness, leucorrhea, spermatorrhea, typhoid and other fevers, coughs and colds.

In leucorrhea and gonorrhea, uterine tonics such as false unicorn or squaw vine (mitchella) may be added. May be taken in infusion or decoction, 1 oz. to 1 pt.

For coughs and colds, add syrup of black cohosh.

Pipsissiwa can be taken by infusion or decoction, 1 oz. to 1 pt.

boiling water in doses of 1 wine-glassful or as required. The Fl. X is more astringent than the infusion.

Pipsissiwa may be used in place of uva ursi.

PLANTAIN (*Plantago Major*)

Although a native of Europe, plantain grows abundantly over most of the U.S.

The taste is astringent with no odor.

It is an old remedy for the poisonous bites and stings of insects and snakes. An immediate application of rubbed leaves or the juice would be useful. Apply also to nettle stings and minor wounds.

Both the ROOTS and LEAVES influence the glandular system and the entire mucous membrane, but especially that of the urinary tract and manifests some useful influence in eczema, scrofula, and strumas. Also in kidney and bladder troubles, aching in the lumbar region, scanty and scalding urine, cystic catarrh, internal and external scrofulous swelling, diarrhea, and as an ointment for irritated piles.

Plantain is also famous as an external application for boils, tumors, and inflammations. A fomentation or a wash of the herb is useful in sprains, erysipelas, ophthalmia, and other surface irritations.

For frog or thrush in children, the following is recommended: 1 oz. plantain seeds boiled in 1½ pts. water down to 1 pt. Strain and sweeten with honey. Take in T. doses 3 or 4 times daily.

Plantain has been used successfully in blood poisoning as an external application.

Plantain leaves in peach seed oil or petroleum jelly stops formation of impetigo and relieves skin inflammation.

Plantain roots, stems, leaves, and seeds, may be used in infusion, decoction, or syrup. The infusion of 1 oz. to 1 pt. boiling water is taken in wine-glassful doses.

PLEURISY ROOT (*Asclepias Tuberosa*)

Pleurisy root is a native of the U.S. and is most abundant in the southern states. Its brilliant orange flowers attract butterflies, therefore the name also given to it is butterfly-weed. It has been called America's finest wild flower.

The ROOT is the only part used in medicine. When dried it is easily pulverized and has a bitter but not otherwise unpleasant taste. It yields its virtues readily to boiling water.

As the name implies, pleurisy rt. is a most valuable remedy in this disease, in which it mitigates the pain and relieves the difficulty in breathing.

It has long been popular in chest and lung troubles such as bronchitis, asthma, chronic cough, acute catarrh, pneumonia, consumption, pleuritis, peritonitis, membranous croup, colds and other pectoral affections, and is especially recommended in pulmonic catarrh. It is particularly helpful in the early stages. It exerts a specific action on the lungs, assisting expectoration and subduing inflammation. It is considered a near-specific in measles and has been used advantageously in acute rheumatism. In eruptive diseases, add ginger or cayenne.

It is said to be gently tonic and has been employed in pains of the stomach arising from flatulance, indigestion, and dysentery.

It influences the skin (sweat glands), the mucous and serous tissues. It influences a flow of blood toward the surface and will relax the capillaries and thereby relieve the heart and arteries of undue tension.

Securing a slow, steady perspiration and gradually easing excessive heat of the skin renders it very serviceable in febrile conditions such as typhus, scarlet, bilious, puerperal, lung and rheumatic fevers where the skin is hot and the pulse rigid.

Excellent in la grippe (influenza) is the following: mix together, all powdered, 2 oz. each pleurisy rt. and golden rod, ½ oz. ginger, 1 dr. capsicum. Give freely in warm infusion in the fever state, using 1 t. to 1 C. hot water. As improvement is shown, add a little more capsicum and decrease the relaxing pleurisy Rt. This is also useful in typhoid and bilious fevers.

A compound very effective in dysmenorrhea and amenorrhea with spasmodic pains is made as follows: 1 oz. pleurisy rt., ½ oz. ea. blue cohosh and wild yam and ¼ oz. ginger. If powders are used, give in warm infusion using 1 t. to 1 C. hot water. If the herbs are used, use 1 oz. of the mixture to 1 pt. boiling water. Cover and keep warm. Take in wine-glassful doses every few hours. It is anti-spasmodic and will stimulate the menstrual flow.

When there is a tendency to decay or slough, pleurisy root is NOT the proper remedy to be used. It is useful in tonsilitis rather than diptheria; in feverish and inflamed conditions rather than in congestions and in cases possessing a stenic rather than an asthenic pulse.

Do NOT use pleurisy root where the skin is cold and the pulse is weak. A more stimulating remedy is called for in such conditions.

A fine preparation for fevers, either in children or adults, is made as follows: mix together 2 oz. powdered pleurisy Rt. and ½ oz. ginger. For an adult use 1 t. to 1 C. hot water. Cover and allow to stand awhile. Drink warm, leaving the sediment. If more stimulation is needed, add a small portion of capsicum.

In large doses, it is often cathartic.

POKE (*Phytolacca Decandra*)

Poke is a native of the U.S. and grows abundantly throughout the states. The young shoots and leaves are much used as food early in the spring boiled like spinach.

The leaves, berries and the root are used in medicine; the BERRIES and the ROOT are official. The root should be dug up late in November. It abounds most in the active principle of the plant, but the berries are milder in action. As its virtues diminish by keeping, a new supply should be procured every year. The leaves should be gathered when the footstalks begin to redden, just previous to the ripening of the berries. The berries should be collected when perfectly ripe.

The berries have little odor, but the taste is slightly sweetish and at first mild, but followed by a sense of acrimony. The active matter is imparted to boiling water and alcohol.

The berries are a relaxing and stimulating alterative influencing the mucous, serous, and glandular structures.

Cook the berries till they burst and pour off the juice without straining. Then cover the berries again with water and cook thoroughly. Now strain off all the juice and boil down to the consistency of a thick syrup and add the first juice poured off. Bottle for use.

It can be made into a tincture with 30% alcohol. This is excellent for rheumatism.

In the treatment of scrofula, it relieves the glandular system of its impurities and cleanses the blood current, increases the flow of saliva, urine, or perspiration, and frees the alvine canal.

In acute and chronic rheumatism, use the following: 1 oz. poke berries, ½ oz. each of elix. wood betony and black cohosh.

The dried root is considered of little value. The root in its green state is quite acrid and irritating to the mucous membrane, frequently causing a persistent vomiting. A similar result will follow if the green root is bruised and placed upon the surface of an excoriated or ulcerated part.

The better way to use poke is to cut the green root fine, cover with boiling water and allow to boil 2 or 3 min. This preparation may be taken in doses of 1 t. to 1 T. with but little, if any, nausea experienced. 2 oz. of alcohol to the pint may be added to keep this preparation. The cooking largely dissipates the nauseating tendency so that much more of it can be taken than of the green root. But only cook 2 or 3 min., it is then a better nervine, alterative, and laxative.

In small doses, it acts as an alterative and has been highly recommended and successfully used in the treatment of chronic rheumatism. It is useful in those forms of rheumatism which attack the synovial membranes (membranes secreting fluid and lining joints) and the ligamentous (tissues holding organs in place) structures. Like many alteratives, it is somewhat slow in action, persistence and time must be given for its influence to manifest.

Poke root is one of the most powerful alteratives. Because it manifests quite a powerful influence upon the glandular structures, it has been largely used in the treatment of hard, enlarged, and swollen glands. It is reliable in skin diseases, used both internally and externally.

Poke root is considered a valuable remedy in dyspepsia, also in treatment of ulcers, ringworm, scabies, grandular conjunctivitis, and dysmenorrhea.

The roasted root forms a good poultice for inflamed surfaces. It quickly reduces excessive suppuration.

A strong infusion of the leaves and roots has been recommended in piles.

An ointment prepared by mixing 1 dr. of the powdered root or leaves with an oz. of lard has been used in psora, any of the various contagious skin diseases, fungus infection of the scalp and hair caused by several species of ringworm, and some other forms of cutaneous diseases. It occasions, at first, a sense of heat and smarting in the part to which it is applied.

An extract is made by evaporating the expressed juice of the recent leaves and has been used for the same purpose.

The following is recommended in the treatment of goiter: all in Fl. X, 3 Dr. poke berries, 2 Dr. cascara sagrada, ½ Dr. ginger in 4 oz. simple syrup.

The FE poke root is a good alterant and, if taken internally for some time with external applications of the bruised green root, it will relieve many a bony and cartilaginous swelling, including bunions. It is claimed that it will avert white swelling.

The Fl. X relieves neuralgia, sciatica, lumbago, and rheumatism.

The Fl. X may be used internally and locally in hot fomentation or poultice. Poke influences all the deep structures when inflamed and all the serous structures. It is a good poultice in case of felon.

The simple infusion is made of 1 T. root, leaves, or berries, cut small steeped in 1 pint boiling water. Take 1 t. as required. The dose of the powdered root, as an emetic, is from 10 to 30 grs., as an alterative from 1 to 5 gr.

The following is a good formula for the compound poke liniment: Fl. X green poke rt. 3 oz., pulv. borax. 1 dr., oil of sassafras 1 dr., oil of bay (laurel) ½ dr. Mix well together, then add a thick mucilage of gum tragacanth sufficient to make 6 oz. Shake well. Apply to parts affected 4 or 5 times daily. Use plenty of friction or kneading in the case of enlargements.

POLYPODY ROOT (Polypodium Vulgare)

This fern is common in the woods throughout the U.S. It is also called female fern and brake root.

The root has a sickening-sweet taste and an unpleasant odor. Water extracts its medicinal properties.

The ROOTS and LEAVES are highly valued as an expectorant to the bronchi, in coughs, consumption, chest diseases, catarrh affections, and especially where expectoration is difficult.

It is a safe and gentle laxative for the bowels. Combined with other remedies, it is useful in hepatic troubles.

As an alterative in skin diseases, it is safe and useful.

As an anthelmintic, it is said that a strong decoction will expel worms.

Polypody root may be used in infusion, decoction or substance. The bruised root is generally used.

The infusion is made with ½ oz. crushed root to 1 pt. boiling water, sweetened and taken in teacup doses frequently. The decoction is made by using 1 oz. crushed root to 1 pt. water, simmer about 15 to 20 min.

POMEGRANATE *(Punica Granatum)*

Pomegranates grow wild upon both shores of the Mediterranean and are cultivated in all countries where the climate is sufficiently warm to allow the fruit to ripen, including our gulf states and other warm areas. A large tropical and sub-tropical bush, it is grown for its brilliant orange-red flowers and its large hard-rinded juicy, pulpy fruit about the size of an orange. The fruit ripens in September. It is quite pleasant in flavor.

One of the favorite fruits of ancient mythology, it is claimed. Bacchus, who seduced the Scythian maid, turned her into a pomegranate tree and placed a crown on the fruit to compensate her for the crown he had promised her before her seduction.

Pomegranates are mentioned many times in the Bible. Those of most interest being: Exodus 28:33 and 34 (B.C. 1491)— "Pomegranates of blue, of purple, and of scarlet around the hem (of priest's robe)."

I Kings 7/20—(B.C. 1005)—"And the pomegranates were 200 in a row around about (referring to the building of the House of the Lord)."

Song of Solomon 4/13 (B.C. 1014)—"Thy plants are an orchard of pomegranates with pleasant fruits."

Song of Solomon 7/12 (B.C. 1014) —"Let us get up early to see pomegranates bud forth."

Song of Solomon 8/2 (B.C. 1014)—"I would bring thee into my mother's house; I would cause thee to drink of spiced wine of the juice of my pomegranates."

The art of making wine from pomegranates of which Solomon speaks is still practised in Persia.

The ancient Chinese revered the pomegranates as one of the three blessed fruits. Because of its many seeds, it was their symbol of a large production of progeny and eternal life.

The *Bible Dictionary* claims the pomegranate was the favorite fruit of Egypt and Palestine. It was considered a very refreshing delicacy to dwellers in a hot land.

A syrup made from the seeds is known as grenadine.

Pomegranate is one of the earliest medicines of importance, considered as a specific for expelling either the round, tape, or pin worm and has been used as a vermifuge since the beginning of the Christian era among Arabian and Indian physicians. The bark of the root was recommended by Hippocrates.

The FLOWERS, BARK, and RIND can all be used as a remedy for tapeworm.

The bark of the root has no smell, when chewed it colors the saliva yellow and leaves an astringent taste without any disagreeable bitterness.

It may be administered in powder or decoction, which is preferred. The following method was used by the Negroes of St. Domingo before it was introduced into Europe. Prepare by taking a dose of castor oil and fast the day preceding that on which the remedy is administered. A decoction is prepared by macerating 2 oz. bruised bark in 2 pts. water for 24 hrs. Then boil down to 1 pt. Take ⅓ portion every ½ hr. The 1st and second dosage may produce vomiting but the 3rd remains. Within one hour after the last dose, the patient usually has 3 or 4 stools in which the worm is discharged. Should the bowels not be opened, an injection should be administered. If not successful the first day, repeat. The decoction was followed by a dose of castor oil.

The Dominion College recommends the following—Soak 2 oz. bark in 2 pts. water for 12 hrs., boil down to 1 pt., strain, and take wine-glassful every 2 hrs. until it is all taken. At times, joints of the worm may come away within 1 hr. of the last dose being taken, but sometimes the dose needs to be repeated a few successive mornings. It is good policy to continue for a few days after the joints have ceased to pass.

Before taking this, or any other worm remedy, it is always best to fast for 24 hrs. and take a cathartic to clear the bowels before, and a dose of anti-bilious cathartic taken after.

The flowers are inodorous, having a bitterish, strongly astringent taste, and impart a violet-red color to the saliva. They were used by the ancients to secure a good red dye. They have the same medicinal property and were used for the same purposes as the rind.

The rind of the fruit and the flowers, in the form of decoction, may be given in diarrhea, chronic dysentery, in the excessive and exhaustive sweats of hectic fever, night sweats of phthisis, or simple debility. The decoction is more frequently used as an injection in leucorrhea and as a gargle in sore and irritated throat in the earliest stages or after the inflammatory action has somewhat subsided. The powdered rind has also been recommended in intermittent fever.

The dose of the rind and flowers in powder is 20 to 30 gr. A decoction may be prepared in the proportion of 1 oz. to 1 pt. boiling water given in doses of 1 to 2 fl. oz. Fruit bark 1 to 2 dr.; Fl. X of root bark, ¼ to 2 Dr. May be administered in powder or decoction but the decoction is preferred.

The fruits are made into cooling drinks to quench the thirst and give relief in feverish complaints.

A strong infusion will be useful in ulcers in the mouth and throat, strengthen the gums, and fasten loose teeth.

The rinds of the fruit are used for the tanning of the finest leathers at Cordova, Spain, now known as Cordovan leather.

WHITE POPLAR (Populus Tremuloides)

The white poplar is a common tree in the U.S. It is also called quaking aspen.

The buds, gathered in winter, are very strongly medicinal. The inner bark and the buds are a stimulating tonic alterant.

The INNER BARK of the tree holds a high rank as a really good general tonic, taking the place of Peruvian bark and quinine; continued use has none of the drawbacks of quinine. One can forget that quinine was ever known if they will use this bark in conditions where quinine would be used.

It is possibly one of the best tonics one can use in old age, or in those brought to a low ebb by disease (debility).

It is very good in sub-acute and chronic diarrhea, chronic dysentery, and cholera infantum. It is a tonic not an astringent.

It tones the mucous membrane, is fine in a lax condition of the stomach resulting in digestive weakness, promotes appetite, and relieves indigestion.

It is one of the most effective tonics to the urinary system. The kidneys and bladder feel its power. In incontinence of urine, it will gradually increase the urine and relieve the aching back. In stricture, and catarrh of the bladder, it is very frequently used. Combined with uva ursi in excess, it will give good results in cystic and renal catarrh and congestions.

In eczema, purulent ophthalmia, syphilitic sores, and chronic gonorrhea, it is an excellent wash. It can be combined with other remedies, and it will not disappoint if a tonic effect is required. Use it in dysuria, and in stranguria.

The famous spiced bitters are made as follows: poplar, barberry bark, and balmony, all in powder and in equal parts. Mix 1 t. powder to 1 C. hot water, sweetened. Drink warm leaving the sediment. This is a fine hepatic tonic and is good for all sluggish conditions of the stomach with biliousness and torpid bowels.

The powder may be filled into capsules and taken in substance instead of the infusion, if desired.

It is also of use as a remedy in the debility of the female generative system; uterine, vaginal, and anal weakness, leucorrhea, and painful menstruation, both as a wash and for internal use.

An injection for anal prolapsus is made by mixing ½ oz. each poplar and bayberry in 16 oz. water.

In all cases of debility, faintness, and hysteria, white poplar bark can be freely taken.

Excellent as an external wash for cuts, bruises, burns, and fetid prespiration.

A simple infusion is made of 1 t. leaves, buds, or bark steeped in 1 C. boiling water. Drink cold 1 or 2 C. daily. When used as a wash, 1 t. borax added to 1 C. tea will be of benefit.

QUEEN'S DELIGHT (Stillingia Sylvatica)

This plant is a native of the U.S. and grows in the pine barrens from Virginia to Florida. When wounded, it emits a milky juice.

The ROOT is the part used. The taste is bitter, acrid, and pungent; the odor is unpleasant. It should be used after being gathered as age impairs its medicinal property. It yields its virtues to water.

It is a good alterative and is useful in obstinate cutaneous affections, skin diseases, eruptions, rheumatism, scrofula, impure conditions of the blood, ulcers, scurvy, syphilis, secondary syphilis, and eczema either in infusion or decoction but usually in combination with remedies of less stimulating nature. It is best adapted to chronic cases.

It has a stimulating influence upon the alvine mucous membrane and the glandular system. It can be taken where a stimulant is needed for the liver and in some cases of constipation, it is of value.

A good liniment for sore throat is made as follows: all in oil, queen's delight and lobelia 2 Dr. each, cajuput and eucalyptus 3 Dr. each, alcohol 3 oz.

In large doses, queen's delight is emetic and cathartic. The oil should NEVER be used internally.

The simple infusion is made of 1 t. root infused in 1 C. boiling water. Drink 1 C. cold tea during the day.

RED RASPBERRY *(Rubus Strigosus)*

This plant needs no introduction as it is quite common. It is extensively cultivated as well as growing wild in many places. It belongs to the rose family.

Unfortunately the medicinal value of raspberry leaves is not sufficiently understood by the masses of people.

The LEAVES and the BARK OF THE ROOT are the parts used medically. They impart their medicinal properties to water. The taste is astringent with no odor. The fruit has a rich, delicious flavor.

Raspberry leaf tea is mild and may, with perfect safety, be given to children in stomach complaints, sweetened with honey or sugar.

The infusion of 1 oz. in 1 pt. boiling water is most effective in removing canker from and toning the mucous membrane. Also for ulcers and wounds. In ophthalmia, the infusion is a first class wash.

For a very fine wash and gargle for relaxed sore throat, canker in the mouth, throat, and tongue and spongy gums, use the following: red raspberry leaves and bayberry bark ½ oz. each. Infuse in 1 pt. boiling water, cover till cold, strain and use as required.

Raspberry leaf tea has long been recommended as a drink during the period of pregnancy and at confinement. There would be fewer cases needing instruments and fewer hemorrhages after delivery. It has a splendid influence upon the uterus, will sustain in labor and relieve after-pains, renders easy and speedy parturition, assists milk secretion, and hastens convalescence. A small portion of cayenne or ladies' slipper can be added to the infusion or at the approach of labor. An addition of ¼ t. of composition powder to 1 oz. leaves in 1 pt. boiling water will prove a valuable adjunct. This should always be taken warm, ½ teacupful every hour during labor.

In constipation, the following will be useful—raspberry leaves 1 oz., mt. flax 1½ oz., infuse in 1½ pts. boiling water. Cover till cold. Strain and take 3 T. 3 or 4 times daily. If the lower bowel needs special attention ¼ or ½ oz. butternut bark may be added.

It will allay nausea and is useful in acute and chronic diarrhea and dysentery and in leucorrhea and gonorrhea, either as a tea or by injection. Make an infusion of 1 oz. leaves to 1 pt. boiling water. If drinking the infusion, a little ginger may be added.

A poultice for removing proud flesh and cleansing wounds is made by combining powdered red elm bark with the infusion.

The expressed juice of the fruit is very nourishing in convalescence and for weak stomachs.

Raspberry leaves may be used instead of coffee or tea when the bowels are in a relaxed state.

The simple infusion is made by steeping 1 t. leaves in 1 C. boiling water. Dose of the Fl. X of the leaves is 1 to 2 Dr.

TURKEY RHUBARB, also EAST INDIAN, CHINA, and ENGLISH (*Rheum Palmatum, Official, Rhaponticum,* and others)

It is claimed that all of these species of rhubarb originated from one particular species but the question yet remains unsettled from what precise plant it is derived. All that is known for certain is that it is the ROOT of one or more species of rheum. Their common names have been given them from their port of export.

The *Rheum Palmatum* or Turkey rhubarb is considered official in the U.S. Although the various species are different in appearance, it is claimed their medicinal properties are about the same. The ROOTS are gathered when they are six years old.

The leafstalks of the different species of rheum have a pleasant acid taste and are useful in making tarts and pies.

Rhubarb has a peculiar aromatic odor, bitter, faintly astringent taste, and when chewed tinges the saliva yellow. Its coloring principle is absorbed and may be detected in the urine causing it often to become quite red. This is caused by the alkaline urine acting upon the yellow matter of the root.

Rhubarb yields all its active properties to water and alcohol. By boiling, the virtues of the medicine are diminished. Its most remarkable singularity is the union of a cathartic with an astringent power: the latter of which, however, does not interfere with the former as the purgative effect precedes the astringent. Rhubarb is one of our mildest and safest remedies in this class.

It is a mild stimulating tonic to the liver, gall ducts, and the alvine mucous membrane. It is not unpleasant to the taste and is generally well received by the stomach; in small doses it invigorates the powers of digestion.

Rhubarb cleanses the mucous membrane of viscid matter. In large doses, it is a simple and safe cathartic producing fecal rather than watery discharges; small and frequent doses are a tonic hepatic. Because of its astringent property, it is NOT the remedy to assist in overcoming chronic constipation but is valuable in the treatment of diarrhea, dysentery, and cholera infantum. Heat somewhat increases its astringency.

When the stomach is enfeebled and the bowels relaxed at the same time and a gentle cathartic is required, rhubarb, as a general rule, is preferrable to all others. Hence its use in dyspepsia attended with constipation, in diarrhea even when purging is indicated in the secondary stages of cholera infantum, in chronic dysentery, and in almost all typhoid diseases when fecal matter is accumulated in the intestines or to prevent such an accumulation.

Owing to its tonic properties, it has found much favor in infantile troubles, especially in stomach troubles and looseness of the bowels, weakened digestion, irritation of the alimentary canal; also in diarrhea and dysentery, rhubarb is especially useful as a laxative, because of its mildness and tonic qualities.

As a general rule, rhubarb is not applicable to cases attended with much inflammatory action. Its griping may be counteracted by adding some aromatic or bicarbonate of soda to relieve the acidity.

The *New England Homestead of 1957* states—"Boiling leaves of the rhubarb in water will brighten aluminum pans that are dark and discolored, without scrubbing or scouring."

The purgative properties of rhubarb are diminished by roasting while its astringency remains unaffected. For this reason, this method has been used in cases of diarrhea. By long boiling, the same effect is produced.

The dose of rhubarb as a purgative is from 20 to 30 gr. As a laxative and stomachic, 5 to 10 gr. The infusion is much used in cases of delicate stomach and is peculiarly adapted to children. The tincture or syrup is also highly useful. The tincture is chiefly used but the powder is effective and reliable. The tincture dose is 5 to 20 min. The simple infusion is made by steeping 1 t. cut root in 1 C. boiling water. Drink cold, 1 C. during the day.

The infusion is of a dark, reddish-yellow color.

COMMON GARDEN RUE *(Ruta Graveolens)*

A native of Southern Europe, the common garden rue is now cultivated in our gardens.

The whole herbaceous part of the plant is active medicinally but the LEAVES are usually employed. These have a strong disagreeable odor, especially when rubbed. Their taste is bitter, hot, and acrid. In the fresh state, they have much acrimony which is diminished on drying. Their virtues depend chiefly on a volatile oil, which is very abundant and apparent over the whole surface of the plant. Both alcohol and water extract their active properties.

From early days rue has been used as a household remedy. The warm infusion made with 1 oz. to 1 pt. boiling water, taken in wine-glassful doses every 1 or 2 hrs. is very effective as a stimulant and tonic upon the uterus; it relieves congestion or suppression of the menses (amenorrhea). May be sweetened with sugar or honey, if desired.

Rue excites the circulation, increasing secretions, especially when they are deficient from debility. Also useful in hysterical affections, gas pains, flatulence, colic, worms, and convulsions in children and adults. Can be given to infants, sweetened with honey, for thrush and canker in the stomach. Do NOT take until 1 hr. after meals. NEVER boil rue.

Ancients used rue as a condiment and believed that it resisted the action of poisons. It is claimed that during the time of the plague, sprigs of rue were carried in the hands as a disinfectant.

Rue is also called *"ave-grace* (herb of grace). It is claimed it is so called by a religious order because it was used in the holy water when sprinkled on the heads of sinners.

Rue is mentioned only once in the Holy Bible: Luke 11/42 (A.D. 33) "For ye tithe mint and rue and all manner of herbs."

The dose of the powder is from 15 to 30 gr. (1 oz), 2 or 3 times a day; the Fl. X is ½ to 1 Dr.; the oil 2 to 5 min. The simple infusion is made by steeping 1 t. herb in 1 C. boiling water.

Rue should not be taken in large doses.

GARDEN SAGE *(Salvia Officinalis)*

The botanical name is derived from *salvare*—meaning "to save"—referring to its great curative and healing power. It was highly esteemed by the ancients and regarded as a panacea for all diseases. It became so popular that it was universally drunk as we drink tea today, as a spring tonic.

Sage grows wild in the South of Europe, but is cultivated abundantly in our gardens. It is one of our most popular plants. It has terminal spikes of blue, light purple, or red blossoms, but all possess the same medical properties. The LEAVES are the official portion.

Both the leaves and the flowering summits have a strong fragrant odor and a warm, bitterish, aromatic, somewhat astringent taste. It imparts its virtues to boiling water in infusion but more especially to alcohol. They abound in a volatile oil which, when distilled, is strongly antiseptic.

In infusion, it may be given in debilitated conditions of the stomach, attended with flatulence, and is said to have been useful in checking the exhaustive sweats of hectic fever. Its most usual application is as a gargle in sore and inflamed throat, mouth ulcers, and the relaxation of the uvula.

A gargle in sore throat and mouth ulcers is made as follows: steep 1 oz. sage, 1 Dr. powdered borax and 2 oz. honey in 1 pint hot (not boiling) water. Cover till cold. Strain and gargle freely. If a more stimulating gargle is desired, equal parts of vinegar and water may be used. Bring to a boil and pour on the ingredients. Cover closely until cold, strain, and use freely.

Another excellent gargle for relaxed throat, quinsy, laryngitis, and tonsils, and also for mouth and throat ulcers is made by pouring ½ pt. hot cider vinegar upon 1 oz. leaves and add ½ pt. cold water. Dose—Drink wineglassful frequently as well as gargle.

The infusion is prepared by macerating 1 oz. of the leaves in 1 pt. boiling water, of which 2 fl. oz. may be taken at once. When intended to be used merely as a pleasant drink in febrile complaints, or to allay nausea, the maceration should continue but a very short time so that all the bitterness (tonic) of the leaves may not be extracted.

It is very soothing to the nerves, being used largely to quiet cerebral nervous excitement and the delirium of fevers. Make the infusion of ½ oz. to 1 pt. of hot or boiling water.

Sage tea taken in cold infusion will, within a few days, cause milk to leave the breasts and prevent milk from forming where this is desirable in nursing mothers, as in the cases of inflammation or gathering in the breasts.

Sage has a marked effect on the brain and the head. It strengthens the sinews and has been used with success in palsy.

It was formerly made into wine and pressed into cheese; also made into stuffing for fowl and sausages and in the 18th century, sage butter was one of the Church's great fasting dishes. Sage is one of the most important herbs for seasoning food, both the red and green-leafed sage being used. The dried and the fresh whole leaves are used. Sage cheese is still sold in our food shops today.

America cannot cultivate enough sage for home consumption and annually imports thousands of tons.

"The use of sage in the month of May, with butter, parsley, and some salt, was considered excellent for continued good health."

In making the infusion, see to it that no steam escapes, as the result will not be nearly as good. The leaves of sage contain considerable volatile oil, hence it should NEVER be boiled.

WILD MEADOW SAGE (Salvia Lyrata)

Also known as "cancer weed," it is considered effective as a poultice in glandular swellings, and warts.

SASSAFRAS (Sassafras Officinale)

Sassafras is common throughout the U.S. Almost all parts are aromatic.

The ROOT BARK and the BARK of the TREE is mostly

used. The woody root is usually sold in the form of chips. The pith in the young shoots (the spongy part) abounds in a gummy matter which it readily imparts to water, forming a limpid mucilage. Gather the pith in the spring and allow to dry.

The root bark is the most popular. The odor is highly fragrant; its taste sweetish and gratefully aromatic. Its medicinal properties are extracted by water and alcohol.

It is most convenient in the form of an infusion and drunk instead of coffee and tea. This is the popular spring tonic. Pick in the spring when the bark has the greatest strength.

It has been particularly recommended as an alterative in rheumatism, especially chronic, gout, skin eruptions, scrofula, scorbutic and syphilitic affections.

Sassafras influences the glandular system and has some reputation in varicose ulcers. Also used as an aromatic in spasms and pains in the region of the heart. In these latter cases, it must be given in warm infusion.

A volatile oil is distilled from the root bark. It is used for scabies and other contagious eruptions. It is a good stimulant for bruises, congestions, inflammations, rheumatism and neuralgic swellings. It is often used to relieve toothache.

A good stimulating liniment is made as follows: all oil, sassafras, cloves, cinnamon, of equal parts.

A poultice of the infusion, with added red elm, is valuable for all sores, bruises, congested swellings, chronic abscesses, ulcers, etc. Drink the infusion at the same time.

Sassafras chips are also used to quite an extent.

SKULLCAP *(Scutellaria Lateriflora)*

Skullcap is one of the finest nervines and antispasmodics ever discovered. It grows in damp places over most of the eastern half of the U.S.

The WHOLE PLANT is used. The taste is somewhat bitter but will not nauseate. It may be used wherever disorders of the nervous system exist. It will be found fully as stimulating to the nerves as the quinine of the medical world without the unpleasant after-effects of that drug.

Its chief influence is spent upon the nervous system, its stimulation of the spinal cord, brain, and sympathetic nervous system bringing to all a tonic influence which is quite permanent.

It gives excellent service in general nervousness, nervous prostration, hysteria, chorea, delirium tremens, convulsions, puerperal convulsions, and other spasmodic conditions of infant or adult, rickets, insomnnia, convalescence from fevers, cranial, facial neuralgia, nervous forms of dyspepsia, seminal weakness, general female weakness, and hypochondria. An addition of lobelia and capsicum or ladies' slipper and cayenne or with blue cohosh alone forms an excellent antispasmodic.

In the delirium of fevers and of typhoid and nervous headache, use an infusion 4 times daily.

In restless and wakeful conditions and when a morphia victim is seeking to break the drug habit, skullcap is very useful. It tones and soothes the nervous system, without any narcotic properties, and often brings on natural sleep. Drink a wine-glassful of infusion 4 times daily.

It has been regarded as a specific in St. Vitus dance (chorea). Skullcap will be helpful in cases of epilepsy.

A simple infusion is made by using 1 oz. herb to 1 pt. boiling water. Cover to keep in the steam. Take a wine-glassful 4 times daily or ½ or 1 glassful can be taken at night before retiring.

Skullcap can be used in powder, pills, capsules, infusion, or the fluid extract.

If taken in capsules, 2, 3, or 4 capsules may be taken twice, 3 times, or more daily, as required.

A hot infusion is considered more diffusive than the fluid extract.

Skullcap should NEVER be boiled.

SERPENTARIA (*Aristolochia Serpentaria*)

Also called Virginia snake root. It grows throughout the Middle, Southern, and Western States.

Its smell is strong, aromatic, and camphorous with a warm, bitter taste that is also camphorous. The ROOT yields all its virtues to water and alcohol.

Taken in small doses, it is used in dyspeptic troubles promoting the appetite and digestion.

In nettle rash or sumac poisoning, take the infusion freely for a few hours, then stop.

It is useful in rheumatism, typhus, and in fevers, especially in typhoid, whether idiopathic or symptomatic, when the system begins to feel the necessity for support but is unable to bear active stimulation. It is accepted by the digestive organs when Peruvian Bark cannot be taken.

In languid or sluggish conditions of the alvine canal, small doses will do good. It is NOT to be used if the alvine canal is irritated.

In infusion, it is useful in all eruptive diseases where the eruption is tardy or has receded; as a gargle in sore or inflamed throat and in malignant sore throat. Also during parturition where the extremities are cold, circulation poor and pains inefficient, and will also prohibit possible flooding. It has been highly recommended in intermittent fevers, though generally inadequate to cure, it has often proven serviceable as an adjunct to Peruvian bark or quinine.

In hot infusion, its influence is primarily toward the skin, the capillaries, and soon it is felt by the whole arterial system and the heart impulse becomes stronger and fuller. By its stimulating action upon the arterial side of the circulation, the whole nervous system is aroused.

The uterus feels its influence, and it is valuable in menstruation suppressed by colds.

A cold infusion quite freely influences the kidneys and relieves congestion and torpor.

Serpentaria should NOT be boiled, as boiling impairs its strength. To do good, take in small doses, use thoroughly and then stop. If an emetic is desired, take in stronger doses.

The general dose of the powdered root is from 10 to 30 gr. or for an infusion, steep 1 t. granulated root in 1 C. boiling water for ½ hr. Take 1 T. 3 to 6 times daily.

The infusion is preferred. The decoction or extract would be less desirable as the volatile oil, upon which the virtues of the medicine partly depend, is dissipated by boiling.

SKUNK CABBAGE *(Symplocarpus Foetidus)*

The skunk cabbage is a very curious plant; the only one of the genus to which it belongs. It is a native of the U.S., growing in wet places.

The ROOT has been employed in medicine for hundreds of years. All parts of it have an extremely disagreeable fetid odor, thought to resemble that of the offensive animal after which it is named. It resides in an extremely volatile principle which is rapidly dissipated by heat and diminished by desiccation. This fetid odor remains, to a greater or less extent, for a considerable period after the completion of the drying process.

The taste, though less decided than in the fresh state, is still acrid, manifesting itself after the root has been chewed for a short time, by a prickling and smarting sensation in the mouth and throat. The acrimony, however, is dissipated by heat and is entirely lost in the decoction. It is also diminished by time and exposure; the root should not be kept for use longer than a single season.

Water or alcohol extracts its virtues.

Skunk cabbage has an enviable reputation in pulmonary consumption. It has been highly recommended in asthma, chronic catarrh, dropsy, chronic rheumatism, hysteria, bronchitis, pleurisy, irritable coughs, whooping coughs, restlessness of fevers and nasal catarrh. Its expectorant, anti-spasmodic, and nervine properties are manifested in these conditions. It is particularly useful in spasmodic asthma.

It may be used in pill form, powder, infusion, or decoction. It is best taken in powder mixed with honey; ½ oz. to about 4 oz. of the honey taken in ½ to 1 t. doses in bronchial and asthmatic cases. In large doses, it occasions nausea and vomiting.

Externally, skunk cabbage, in the form of an ointment, has a soothing effect.

SPEARMINT *(Mentha Viridis)*

Spearmint is a native of England. It now grows wild in many parts of the U.S. and is cultivated in gardens for domestic use. It is also grown extensively for its oil.

Spearmint is often just called mint. The odor is strong and aromatic; the taste warm and slightly bitter, less pungent than that of peppermint and is considered by some as more agreeable. These properties are retained for some time by the dried plant. They depend on a volatile oil which is imparted to alcohol and water by maceration.

Being one of the mint family, it should NOT be boiled, as it is very volatile.

It may be used in warm infusion where a mild perspiration is desired.

It is unlike peppermint in that it also possesses diuretic properties and is suitable in inflammation of the kidneys and bladder and in suppression of the urine, it induces free discharge of the watery portion of the urine.

It has always held a foremost place in vomiting, in allaying sickness at the stomach and nausea by taking a weak warm infusion. The vomiting of pregnancy will often yield to it, and it readily quiets the stomach after emesis. Persistent vomiting in pregnancy can often be helped by the following: ½ oz. spearmint, 2 Dr. each cloves, cinnamon and rhubarb infused in 1 pt. boiling water. Cover for 20 min., strain and take a wine-glassful (3 or 4 T.) every 30 min. May be sweetened with sugar, if desired. In colic, flatulence and hysteria, add 1 part ginger to 3 parts spearmint infusion.

For hay asthma, the following is an excellent preparation: mix well equal parts of oil of peppermint and oil of spearmint in vaseline. Apply up the nostrils with a pencil brush or atomizer. It is also useful in catarrh conditions. It is soothing and healing to the mucous membranes and will protect them from the irritation of cold air.

As a liniment applied to various aches and pains, the following is useful: 1 part each of oil of spearmint and oil of rosemary and 10 parts of Tr. lobelia.

Wash the hands and heads of children with a decoction of spearmint when they are suffering from scabs.

The oil may be used for the same purpose as the herb. May be sweetened for internal use. For infantile troubles, the sweetened infusion is an excellent remedy.

The usual infusion is made up of 1 oz. in 1 pt. boiling water, taken in doses of a wine-glassful.

It is claimed that the Greeks and Romans used spearmint as a relish in most dishes. Perhaps that is the reason mint sauce is so popular (see Peppermint for recipe).

Bible quotes are as follows: Matthew 23/23—"Ye pay tithe of mint and anise and cummin."

Luke 11/42—"Ye tithe mint and rue and all manner of herbs."

SUMACH (Rhus Glabra)

Variously called smooth sumach, Pennsylvania sumach, and

upland sumach, this shrub is found in almost all parts of the U.S.

The bark and the leaves are astringent, but the official parts are the BARK and the BERRIES. Both yield their active influence to water.

The red berries have a sour, astringent, not unpleasant taste and are often eaten by the country people. An infusion of the berries has been recommended as a cooling drink in febrile complaints and as a pleasant gargle in inflamed, sore and ulcerated throat. To prepare the drink, cover a quantity of the berries with boiling water and allow to infuse about ½ hr. Strain and sweeten to taste. Also useful in irritated conditions of the bladder, in the treatment of diabetics, and in the relief of bloody urine. Mixed with fresh pineapple juice, it is a most useful gargle in diphtheria and sore throat.

An infusion of the inner bark of the root used as a gargle is considered almost as a specific in the sore mouth attending inordinate mercurial salivation.

In relaxed bowel conditions, chronic diarrhea, intestinal and rectal hemorrhage, and in inflammation of the bladder, the bark is often used as it is more stimulating and tonic.

It is a good wash for aphthous sore mouth and spongy gums.

In prolapsed uterus and prolapsus ani, using an infusion of the bark, either by drinking or as an injection, might be helpful.

As an injection in leucorrhea, the leaves prepared in infusion are equal to witch hazel, having the same soothing influence but being more drying. Prepare the infusion by steeping 1 oz. of the leaves in 1 pt. boiling water. As the leaves are the least astringent, they are valuable in dysentery and hemorrhage of the lungs and uterus.

The decoction is made with 1 oz. bark to 1 pt. boiling water. It is used in doses of 1 wine-glassful or more internally or externally.

NOTE—There are several species of sumach which possess poisonous properties. If the reader decides to pick the berries, be sure you have the right sumach.

TANSY *(Tenacetum Vulgare)*

Tansy is an old world plant now naturalized and growing all over the U.S. It is often grown in the herb garden for medicinal purposes and occasionally for flavoring. The name "tansy" is presumed to come from the Greek name Athanasia meaning "immortality" or "everlasting."

In the old days, tansy was a very popular herb. It was used in Easter cakes and puddings, because it was considered good for the health in the springtime.

As a flavoring, it is used in omelets, baked, and fried fish, etc. The liquor, Chartreuse, is made from it.

It is also used in closets to repel moths, and it is claimed that meat wrapped or rubbed with the leaves will keep the flies away (this should be of interest to campers).

The entire HERB is official in the U.S.

The odor is strong, peculiar, and fragrant but much diminished by drying. The taste is warm, bitter, somewhat acrid, and aromatic. These properties are imparted to water and alcohol. The medical virtues of the plant depend on a bitter extractive and a volatile oil. The seeds contain the largest proportion of the bitter principle and the least of the volatile oil. They must be cut in full bloom, dried carefully, and stored in a tightly closed container.

Tansy has the medicinal properties common to the aromatic bitters and has been recommended as a tonic in intermittents, female conditions such as hysteria, kidney weakness, ammenorrhea, and as a preventative of severe temporary attacks of arthritis, after exhaustive diseases (debility) and fevers. As a tonic, an infusion is said to soothe the nerves and aid digestion. It is recommended for palsy because of its good effect on the sinews.

A hot infusion will influence a free outward flow of circulation, useful for the relief of colds, menstrual flow when suppressed by a recent cold, and in painful menstruation.

In palpitation, boil 1 oz. in 1 pt. water for 10 min. and take 1 wine-glassful 4 or 5 times daily. The results will be excellent.

Tansy is often used as a reliable remedy for worms. The seeds are said to be most effectual. The dose of the powder is from 30 gr. to a dr., 2 or 3 times a day but the infusion is used more frequently. The infusion of 1 oz. to 1 pt. boiling water is taken warm in ½ teacupful doses, night and morning, fasting, for a few days. This should expel both thread and tapeworms in children and adults. Give children ½ that quantity.

A decoction of tansy is a good foment for sprains and a poultice will frequently relieve pruritis vulva.

Tansy flowers are fine for winter bouquets. Cut flowers when freshly opened and dry.

An excellent green dye is made from the roots.

Dose of the Liq. X, ½ to 2 Dr.

Tansy must NOT be used by the pregnant, especially the oil.

BLESSED OR HOLY THISTLE (Carbenia Benedicta)

The blessed thistle is a native of Europe, now cultivated in gardens all over the world. It is now naturalized in the U.S.

It has a feeble, unpleasant odor and an intensely bitter taste, more disagreeable in the fresh than the dried plant. Water and alcohol extract its virtues. The infusion formed with cold water is a grateful bitter; the decoction is nauseous and offensive to the stomach. The bitterness remains in the extract. The whole HERB is used.

The cold infusion, made of ½ oz. LEAVES to 1 pt. water is a mild tonic in weak and debilitated conditions of the stomach, biliousness, excellent in dyspepsia, remitting and intermitting fevers, and loss of appetite. The dose of the powder as a tonic is 1 dr.; that of the infusion is 2 fl. oz.

The warm infusion, 1 oz. to 1 pt. boiling water, in wine-glassful doses will be found of value in breaking up colds; also in menstrual derangements due to colds.

The warm infusion of the leaves is a relaxing diaphoretic, producing only mild perspiration.

A stronger infusion, taken warm while confined to bed, produces copious perspiration.

A still stronger infusion or the decoction, taken in large doses, promotes nausea and vomiting without pain and inconvenience, its influence being manifested upon the liver and gall ducts, the results being a free flow of bile.

For females with pelvis weakness and constipation, add 2 parts squaw vine (mitchella) to 1 part thistle.

As a clarifier of blood, drinking an infusion once or twice a day, sweetened with honey, it would be useful for headache, or what is commonly called the migraine. In fact, this plant has very great power in the purification and circulation of the blood, from the bad state of which arise all the humors of the body.

It will also cleanse the stomach, which must produce good

blood, and good blood cannot but produce good and healthy secretions.

It is also good for dropsy or ague, neither of which can exist if the circulation of blood be pure. Every mother would do well to give thistle to her daughter from the age of 10 to 20. It may prevent them enduring years of pain and misery.

It strengthens all the principal members of the body as the heart, the stomach, the kidneys, the liver, and the lungs.

There is no doubt about this plant being used for centuries. It is certainly a fine blood medicine, and combined with queen's delight, yellow parilla, or the dock roots (red dock, yellow, or burdock) will form a very useful alterative remedy.

Chamomile may be substituted.

GARDEN THYME *(Thymus Vulgaris)*

This plant is native to South Europe, but is cultivated in many gardens in the U.S.

The Greeks used thyme as incense and strewed the floors of monasteries, churches, and banquet halls, bringing out their delightful scent.

Thyme has a strong, spicy odor and taste. It yields its medical properties to boiling water and alcohol.

Can be used externally in fomentation.

In fever conditions, the warm infusion will promote perspiration. Make an infusion of 1 oz. HERB to 1 pt. boiling water. Cover well and keep warm. Can be taken freely and safely at all ages. When making the infusion see that the container is covered so no steam escapes, otherwise the results will not be satisfactory.

A hot infusion will influence menstruation obstructed by cold, relieve colds, colic, and flatulence.

It is a reliable nervine, and taken freely is considered useful for nightmare, melancholy, and insomnia.

It is useful in throat and bronchial irritation, asthma, and lung troubles.

It is considered a specific for whooping cough. For very young children, a little honey or sugar may be added. Give small but frequent doses.

Thymol is made from the oil extracted from thyme. It is an

antiseptic and is added to many liniments. It has an agreeable odor and is often inhaled in pulmonary troubles and used as a deodorant in sick rooms.

Vinegar of thyme is made by steeping thyme in vinegar until the desired strength is reached; it is also used in this way or inhaled to relieve a nervous headache.

Domestically thyme is a favorite seasoning in many foods.

The flowers are very popular as a delightful addition to sachets and potpourris.

FALSE UNICORN (Chamaelirium Lutem)

Also known as fairy wand, studflower, and falsely called blazing star and devil's bit.

False unicorn grows in the moist woodlands and meadows of the south, east and midland states.

Its taste is bitter and inodorous.

False unicorn ROOT is one of the best and most positive stimulating tonics to the uterus and ovaries. It is also a good general tonic, including the mucous membrane. In cases, where the stomach rejects almost all else, false unicorn will frequently be well received. It is, therefore, useful in pregnancy and gastric troubles.

It is however in uterine troubles that it is most useful, also in prolapsus uteri, barrenness, uterine atony, leucorrhea, relaxed vagina, hemorrhage, excessive menstruation, sterility, threatened miscarriage, and spermatorrhea, weakness of the reproductive organs, or when conditions exist where a stimulating tonic is needed; equally strengthening and toning to the generative organs of either male or female. It has been used with good effects in impotency of the male.

In cases where a pregnancy would NOT be desirable, do NOT use false unicorn. On the other hand, it is excellent as a preventative of miscarriage, even after pain is prominent and hemorrhage has made an appearance.

It is also of service in atony of the kidneys, albuminaria, Bright's disease, diabetes, enuresis, bladder, urethra, and in gleet.

Helonin (Fl X) in 5 to 10 grains doses may be used with much advantage in Bright's disease.

In cases of diabetes, the following will be found very valuable in that it decreases both the quantity of water and of the sugar; equal parts of false unicorn and balmony in infusion and taken as required.

The tonic properties are very useful in the treatment of dyspepsia and for expelling the stomach worm.

As a stimulating expectorant and tonic to the bronchi, add spikenard.

False unicorn is best taken in small doses 3 to 6 times a day, but in cases of threatened miscarriage, Fluid X may be taken in doses of from 5 to 10 drops in water every 15 min. to 1 hr.

The following, it is said, will insure against any unnatural complication during pregnancy and to secure prompt and easy delivery. Take about 2 mos. prior to delivery, if troubled and delicate. If needed, it may be taken more or less all through the pregnancy: take every night, 1 gr. helonin (Fl. X) and ¼ gr. black cohosh.

Helonin (the fluid X) is considered the best preparation and represents the root quite fully.

TRUE UNICORN (*Aletris Farinosa*)

This plant is found in almost all parts of the U.S. growing in fields and about the borders of the woods.

It is intensely bitter, the bitterness being extracted by alcohol. The decoction is moderately bitter, but much less so than the tincture.

In small doses the ROOT appears to be simply tonic and may be used advantageously for similar purposes with other bitters of the same class. The powder may be taken in a dose of 10 grains.

The ROOT is a good general tonic, but is especially useful in female troubles. May be taken in all cases of debility in small doses. In dysmenorrhea, it will assist in restoring normal conditions, easing the pain and toning the uterus. In menorrhagia, it will relieve the excess flow. Much that has been written of false unicorn applies to this article. It may safely be given during the whole of the pregnant state, where called for. It is an excellent and perhaps the best preventative of miscarriage, and is an excellent preparatory parturient.

In sterility, barrenness, and impotence, it has been used with good results, sometimes within a few weeks. In difficult cases, however, it may be continued for some months. In dyspepsia or when the stomach is upse in pregnancy, if taken in small doses twice daily, it will afford relief.

True unicorn is NOT to be used where frequent pregnancy is undesirable. In such cases use squaw vine (mitchella) instead. These two, together, form a good female tonic.

Another good female tonic can be made with 4 oz. ea. true unicorn, black haw bark, and wild yam root, and 1 oz. squaw vine (mitchella). Simmer in 1 qt. water 20 min. Strain and take 2 or 3 T. 3 times daily.

A good nervine tonic in depressed and irritated conditions is made with 2 Dr. ea. of FE true unicorn, FE cramp bark, FE skullcap, and FE wild yam in 4 oz. simple syrup.

UVA URSI (Arctostophylos Uva Ursi)

This hardy shrub grows in great abundance in the northern part of the U.S. It was formerly imported from Europe.

The GREEN LEAVES are the only part used in medicine. The fresh leaves are inodorous but, when dried and powdered, acquire a smell not unlike that of hay. The taste is bitterish, strongly astringent, and ultimately sweetish. Water extracts their active principles which are also soluble in alcohol.

Though known to the ancients, it had passed into almost entire neglect until it was revived about the middle of the last century. It has acquired some reputation as being a preventative of urinary calculus and is undoubtedly serviceable in gravel, probably by giving tone to the digestive organs and preventing the accumulation of principles calculated to produce a secretion or precipitation of calculous matter.

Uva ursi is astringent and tonic and while influencing all the mucous membranes, it specially influences that of the genital and urinary organs. It is possibly without an equal in chronic inflammation of the bladder and kidneys. In chronic nephritis, it is a popular remedy. It is considered a specific in ulceration of the kidneys, bladder, and urinary passages. In practically all the diseases of the urinary organs, this remedy is of real service; incontinence of urine, aching back from kidney troubles, congestion or prostatic weakness. It has been used in combination with other remedies in stranuary with good effect. It increases the flow of urine, relieving the congestion and toning the parts.

In catarrh of the bladder, gleet, gonorrhea, and leucorrhea, the leaves of this plant will be helpful.

A very serviceable remedy for use in gravel, stricture, suppression of urine, catarrh of the bladder, or inflammation, infuse ½ oz. each of uva ursi, white poplar bark, and marshmallow root in 1 pt. boiling water for 20 min. Strain and take 3 T. 3 times daily.

In cases of cystic catarrh, prolapsus uteri, flaccid vagina and uterus, aching of the kidneys and bladder, the following is a good pelvic tonic: 1 oz. each uva ursi and squaw vine (mitchella) and 1½ oz. dandelion root simmered in 1 qt. water 20 min. Strain and take 3 or 4 T. 3 times daily.

In Enuresis, the following is a good formula: 1 oz. uva ursi and ½ oz. each of white poplar, sumach berries, and yarrow. Simmer in 1 qt. water for 20 min. Strain and take 3 T. 3 times daily. Use the hot sitz bath daily or rub the lumbar region every day with a solution of common salt and cold water.

Uva ursi is best in hot infusion, but its tonic effect is best obtained from cold preparations. The decoction is usually preferred.

The simple infusion is made by steeping 1 oz. leaves in 1 pt. boiling water, taking a wine-glassful 3 to 4 times daily. The dose of the powder is from a scruple to a drachm., repeated 3 or 4 times daily.

VALERIAN *(Valerian Officinalis)*

Valerian is a native of Europe but is grown and used in the U.S. The English valerian, however, is considered the best.

The official part is the ROOT. The odor, which in the fresh root is slight, in the dried is strong and, though pleasant to some, is disagreeable to others. It is said to be highly attractive to cats. The taste is, at first, sweetish, afterwards bitter and aromatic. It is often covered by adding essence of anise or lavender.

Valerian yields its medicinal properties to water and alcohol. As the virtue of valerian resides chiefly in the essential oil, it should NEVER be made in decoction and NEVER boiled. It may be taken in powder or infusion, which is preferred.

Valerian is especially directed to the nervous system, but without narcotic effect. It is useful in cases of irregular nervous action when not connected with inflammation or an excited condition of the system.

It is particularly recommended in hysteria, hypochondria, epilepsy, migraine, low forms of fever attended with restlessness, morbid vigilance, all symptoms of nervous derangements, nervous debility, weakness or irritability of the nervous system, insomnia, and the nervousness of children. It allays pain and promotes sleep.

It has also been used in intermittents combined with Peruvian bark.

In cases of children with measles, scarlet fever, and other diseases which make them restless, give small doses of the infusion twice or 3 times daily. A sound sleep will result. The same method is also useful in convulsions of infants. Use the essence of aniseed or lavender to cover the taste in these cases, if needed.

A good compound for convulsions, hysteria, colic, cramps, and dysmenorrhea is the following: 1 oz. ea. of FE valerian, FE wild yam, FE blue cohosh, ess. of aniseed in 6 oz. of syrup of ginger. Take from 1 t. to 1 dessert-spoonful 3 or 4 times daily.

In restlessness, insomnia, hysteria, neuralgia, and similar troubles the following is a good combination: infuse ½ oz. each valerian, skullcap, and mistletoe in 1½ pts. boiling water. Cover and allow to stand 2 hrs. Strain and take 2 to 4 T., 4 times daily.

As an excellent nervine, the following may be taken in powder or capsules or made into an infusion and taken hot or cold: 1 oz. each powdered valerian, powdered ginger, powdered lobelia, and 2 oz. powdered pleurisy root.

A simple nerve tonic is made by pouring 1 pt. boiling water on 1 oz. root. Cover until cold and take 2 T. 3 or 4 times daily.

The tincture is official.

The powder is taken in doses of 30 to 90 gr., 3 or 4 times daily.

VERVAIN *(Verbena Hastata)*

Vervain is a native of the U.S. It grows wild and is also cultivated in many gardens.

The taste is bitter and the odor slightly aromatic, when the HERB is rubbed.

It is a very powerful sweating HERB and as such is advantageously used in the early stages of fever. In coughs and colds, a warm infusion (sweetened if desired) taken at commencement will often drive out all congestion overnight. If the stomach needs a thorough cleaning, a warm infusion of vervain and pennyroyal taken every ½ hr. in ½ C. doses will be serviceable. Stay in bed and keep warm while taking it. Large doses are emetic.

The infusion, taken cold, is said to make a good tonic. A cold preparation of vervain is excellent in convalescence from fevers and other debilitating diseases.

The warm infusion, while manifesting its influence in an increased capillary circulation, will be found very soothing to the nervous system in such nervous troubles as delirium, sleeplessness, nervous headache, fits, and convulsions.

It also has a reputation in worms. Take the juice, with sugar, freely for 3 days.

In sick headache, the following is considered a very fine remedy. Pour 1½ pts. boiling water on ½ oz. each vervain, skullcap, and wahoo bark, and ¼ oz. syrup of ginger. Cover and let stand till cold. Strain and take 2 T. every 3 or 4 hrs. In chronic cases, take 3 times daily for some time.

For spleenitis, mix together elix vervain 2 oz. and 1 oz. each elix. boneset and elix. prickly ash. Take 1 T. every 2 or 3 hrs.

For a good tonic hepatic, mix together ½ oz. each syrup of vervain and syrup of balmony and 1 oz. syrup of prickly ash.

WAHOO *(Euonymus Atropurpureus)*

This shrub grows in many sections of the U.S., mostly in the woods.

The BARK of the root, trunk, and twigs is used, the root bark being the stronger. It has a bitter, acrid taste and is nearly inodorous. It yields its medicinal properties to water and alcohol.

It is the slow, persistent, and reliable laxative qualities that have made wahoo a really valuable remedy. For a cathartic effect in habitual constipation, combine 1 oz. FE wahoo with 4 oz. syrup of butternut; dose, 1 t. morning and evenings or evenings only.

It is a reliable bitter tonic hepatic influencing the liver, both in secreting the bile and also in excreting it from the gall cyst. It will induce a mild but persistent flow of bile. It is principally used for this purpose, and this influence is manifested upon the bowels.

Its tonic influence is extended throughout the mucous membrane. In biliousness, jaundice, chronic constipation, especially if due to inactivity of the liver, and skin troubles where hepatic torpor needs reliable help, wahoo can be used with confidence. It improves the appetite and gastric digestion and slowly but persistently relieves cholaemic poisoning.

It is useful in chronic coughs where a torpid liver is largely at fault. It may be added to cough syrups.

In rheumatism, it is frequently combined with alteratives.

In dropsy, it is best combined with milkweed (bitter rt.) or with some diuretic such as couch grass.

In torpid conditions of the digestive tract, wahoo may be added to alteratives. In dyspepsia, it is tonic to the gastric membrane but should be taken in small quantities and in frequent doses.

For a stimulating hepatic, mix 5 dr. FE wahoo, 2 dr. FE culvers rt. and 3 gr. American mandrake in 6 oz. syrup of ginger, dose, 1 t. once to 3 times daily.

A pleasant hepatic is made by adding 4 parts syrup of ginger to 1 part Fl. X wahoo and take 1 t. twice or 3 times daily.

The concentration "euonymin" is generally used in pill form and in combination with other tonics, laxatives, etc.

WITCH HAZEL (Hamamelis Virginica)

The witch hazel grows over most of the Eastern U.S. For centuries, the shoots of this tree were used as divining rods to discover water and metals underground. It is an old time medical remedy that, we are told, is still popular with the American Indians.

The BARK, LEAVES, and TWIGS are all used in medicine. The taste is astringent and sweetish, and the odor is a feeble fragrance. Water extracts its virtues.

It chiefly influences the mucous membrane.

The distilled or aqueous X is a highly favored remedy for household use. It is preferred as a local application in gonorrhea and gleet. In prolapsus uteri, vaginal catarrh, leucorrhea, and relaxed vagina, it is a good injection. It tones the uterus and vagina. Combined with golden seal, it makes a soothing injection for the urethra.

Either the infusion or the distilled X is of excellent value.

A rectal injection of the X is of service in rectal hemorrhage, in hemorrhoids, piles, and prolapsus ani. For bleeding piles, use an injection made from the decoction of the bark or use a local application of an ointment made by adding 1 part Fl X bark to 9 parts simple ointment.

For itching and irritation of piles, an ointment made with lard and a decoction of white oak bark, apple tree bark, and witch hazel is a valuable remedy.

For varicose or prominent veins, it is highly recommended. Apply a lint bandage and keep it constantly wet with the X.

In dysentery and diarrhea, it may be combined with red elm.

In catarrh of any part of the mucous membrane, it is an excellent remedy. In nasal catarrh, use with an atomizer or mix with vaseline and apply with a camel hair brush up the nostrils. In bleeding from the nose, the X may be snuffed up the nose.

The distilled aqueous X is a very good wash for inflamed eyes, and in purulent ophthalmia, it has a soothing effect on the eyes. It may be diluted with rose water or elder flower water either to bathe, make fomentations, or eye pads.

Use an infusion for sore mouth and gums.

As a wash in scaly or skin diseases, wash with a strong infusion. Will act as a tonic to the skin, relieve inflammation, and remove the red veins.

In conjunctivitis, the following is recommended: distilled witch hazel and aqua camphora each ½ oz., aqua rose 1 oz. Put 2 drops in the eyes 3 times daily.

The infusion made of 1 t. bark or leaves steeped in 1 C. boiling water is taken 1 C. a day.

"Hamamelin," a concentrated form of witch hazel, is useful in the treatment of piles in the form of suppositories.

AMERICAN WORMSEED *(Chenopodium Anthelminticum)*

Also called Jerusalem oak.

An indigenous plant, American wormseed grows in almost all parts of the U.S. but most vigorously and abundantly in the southern states. It is known in New Zealand as California spearmint.

The whole herb has a strong, peculiar, offensive, yet somewhat aromatic odor, which it retains when dried. All parts of the plant are occasionally employed, but the SEEDS only are strictly official. The seeds should be collected in the fall, when they are ripe.

They have a bitterish, somewhat aromatic, pungent taste and are possessed in a high degree of the peculiar smell of the plant. They abound in a volatile oil, upon which their medicinal virtues depend. This oil impregnates, to a greater or lesser extent, the whole plant.

Wormseed is one of our most efficient American anthelmintics, chiefly used to expel intestinal worms. It is particularly adaptable to children. The powdered seeds are taken in doses of 20 to 30 gr. for a child and 1 to 2 dr. for an adult, given in honey, jam, or syrup before breakfast in the morning, or at bedtime in the evening for 3 or 4 days successively, this followed by a brisk cathartic such as senna tea. If the worms are not expelled, the same plan is repeated. The dose for a child 2 or 3 years old is from 1 to 2 scruples.

The seeds are rich in a valuable OIL which is perhaps more frequently given than the seeds in substance, though its offensive odor and taste sometimes render it of difficult administration. The dose for a child is from 5 to 10 drops and an adult 10 to 20 drops on sugar each morning and followed after 3 days by a cathartic. An infusion with milk is also often given in wineglassful doses. As the oil is a strong emmenagogue, it should NOT be used during pregnancy.

An excellent formula for worms is the following: oil of wormseed 30 drops, oil of anise 6 drops, sugar of milk 1 dr. Mix and divide into 6 powders. Take 1 or 2 powders every 3 hrs., followed at night by a cathartic.

An infusion of the LEAVES is a far more pleasant, stimulating, aromatic anthilmintic.

A hot infusion may be used to relieve and increase the menstrual flow in case of cold.

A tablespoon of the expressed juice of the leaves or a wineglassful of a decoction prepared by boiling 1 oz. of the fresh plant in 1 pt. milk, with the addition of orange peel or other aromatic, is sometimes used instead of the ordinary dose of the seeds and oil.

WILD YAM (*Dioscorea Villosa*)

Also known as rheumatism root and colic root.

This is not the same yam people eat like potatoes.

This wild yam is a slender vine growing most profusely in

the tropical portion of the U.S. The taste is insipid, afterwards acrid, and it is inodorous.

It is valuable in all forms of colic, especially in bilious colic and in the pains consequent upon gall stones. It will relieve in a positive manner, relax the muscular fibre, and soothe the nerves.

It is useful in cholera morbus, flatulence, facial neuralgia, and in almost any painful condition, it affords wonderful relief. For uterine pains and for after pains, wild yam cannot be surpassed.

In the pains commonly found in the pregnant state, with nervousness and restlessness, it would be difficult to over-estimate the value of wild yam. It may be taken throughout the whole period of pregnancy with excellent results. It quiets nausea. It is a superior preventative of miscarriage and in the trying cramps in the region of the uterus in the latter stages of pregnancy.

In the preliminary stage of parturition in nervous females, it quiets the nerves and helps in labor.

For the prevention of miscarriage and to ease the pains, the following is excellent: 1 oz. each wild yam, squaw vine (mitchella), and false unicorn and ½ oz. black haw simmered in 1 qt. water for 20 min. Strain and take wine-glassful every 3 or 4 hours.

In dysmenorrhea, make a hot infusion with 3 parts wild yam and 1 part ginger. It will give speedy relief. This will also relieve uterine hyperaemia, produce a good outward flow of blood to the surface and a menstrual flow.

Wild yam is extremely good in nervous excitability. In nervous rheumatism, it soothes, tones, and relaxes.

Sciatica can be helped with wild yam, cramp bark, poke root, and oil of wintergreen.

In abdominal and intestinal irritation, spasms, spasmodic asthma, vomiting, and hepatic congestion, take a decoction of 1 oz. ROOT in 1 pt. water; take in T. doses until relieved.

As a female tonic for cramps, pains, and nerves, the following is excellent: FE wild yam 3 parts, FE cramp bark 1 part, FE squaw vine (mitchella) 4 parts.

YARROW (Achillea Millefolium)

Yarrow is very common in Europe and the U.S. It is most often found on roadsides and waste lands.

In the old days of tournaments, yarrow was called "soldiers

woundwort," because it was the basis of a healing ointment made in every castle and monastery. It was named Achillea to commemorate Achilles, the Greek hero.

While one of the most common wayside herbs, it is without doubt one of the most valuable herbs in the world, having a wide range of uses. It is to be regretted that its value is not better known.

The WHOLE PLANT is used. It possesses a faint, pleasant, peculiar smell and a rather sharp, rough, astringent taste. Alcohol or water will extract its virtues.

The hot infusion, taken freely, will raise the heat of the body, equalizing the circulation and producing perspiration. Most useful in colds, obstructed perspiration, and in the commencement of fevers. It opens the pores freely and purifies the blood. Add elder flowers and peppermint for influenza and colds. It has been used in this form from ancient times. Simply pour 1 pt. boiling water on 1 oz. of the HERB. Cover a few minutes and take freely while warm. Drinking a whole pint of this infusion and with a hot water bottle wrapped in flannel wrung out of vinegar applied to the feet, has abated scores of colds by the next morning. Effective for children as well as adults.

It is useful in measles and all the eruptive diseases, particularly where the eruption is slow in making its appearance. Yarrow can be also used with good effect in dyspepsia, jaundice, piles, mucous discharges from the bladder, and incontinence of urine. For enuresis, take in cold infusion or decoction.

The HERB is most reliable in chronic affections of the mucous surfaces of the internal organs. It stimulates the appetite and tones the digestive organs. It will be found extremely useful in chronic dysentery and diarrhea. When false membranes have formed in the small intestines, yarrow can be relied upon to gradually remove them. In such cases take 2 to 4 oz. of the decoction 3 or 4 times daily 1 hr. before meals. If the bowels are badly constipated, take a good herbal laxative. In preparing the decoction, pour 1 qt. cold water on 1 oz. dried herb or 4 oz. green herb; simmer down to 1 pt., strain and take cold. Persevere, as it sometimes takes a little time.

The following has been used for many years with success in removing false membranes from the intestines and has also been very successfully used in fistula and piles: boil 2 oz. dried yarrow and 1 oz. ginger in 4 qts. water down to 2 qts. Strain and while hot, add 3# best molasses. Take cold in ½ C. doses 4 times daily, before meals.

Where the piles protrude, bathe night and morning with warm water, then apply a little tincture of myrrh, and when this has dried, apply a little chickweed ointment. With hemorrhage and pains in the sacral region, the above remedy is splendid and will bring away quantities of false membrane.

In typhoid fever, yarrow is a most desirable remedy because it will not irritate the condition. Its influence will be manifest in regulating the functions of the liver, favorably influencing the secretions throughout the whole alimentary canal; the mucous membrane of the stomach and bowels will be assisted, and the glandular system will also feel its sanative effect. The skin will become soft and moist, the arterial excitement, so common in this condition, will be quieted and sleep will be natural.

In typhoid or other fevers, take 2 or 3 fl. oz. of the decoction every 2 or 3 hrs. as necessary. If a laxative is called for, take a tea made of mt. flax occasionally until the desired result is obtained.

In the spitting of blood and hemorrhages, use the warm infusion. The slow elevation of temperature and production of steady perspiration relieves the pressure from the ruptured vessel, thus relieving the hemorrhage and allowing the vessel to heal.

In cold infusion, it is serviceable in leucorrhea and inflammation of the bladder.

A good combination in febrile conditions is the following: pour 1 qt. water on 1 oz. yarrow and 1 oz. angelica, simmer to 1 pt., strain and take cold, 2 fl. oz. every 2 hrs.

Yarrow is a good tonic to use after worms are expelled. It is of much importance as a tonic to the general system. Combined with uterine tonics, its influence will be felt upon the generative organs and will be serviceable in gleet and vaginal laxity.

In cold infusion, it is useful as a tonic in convalescence from fevers, from nervous prostration, and in phthisis and night sweats.

Although this book was meant to be an all-American Herbal, I thought it necessary to include a number of foreign remedies that are very familiar and popular with many people.

ALOES *(Socotrine, Barbadoes, and Cape Aloes)*

Aloes was well-known to the ancients and much used as a medicine in the tropics where they are grown. Although socotrine originates from East Africa, barbadoes from the West Indies, and cape aloes from South Africa, they are all used for the same purpose.

Socotrine is considered the best and most expensive, the cape aloes, the most abundant and cheapest.

They have a peculiar, not unpleasant odor, and the taste, though bitter and disagreeable, is accompanied by an aromatic flavor.

The LEAVES furnish a juice which, when expressed and evaporated, gives us the aloes of commerce. It is used fresh and dehydrated. Aloes, taken in the liquid state, produce the same effect as when taken in pill or powder, except that in the liquid form it acts more speedily.

They are all cathartic, operating very slowly but certainly, and all have a stimulating effect on the large intestines and the alvine mucous membrane. The discharge is seldom very thin or watery. Aloes are NOT suited to irritated or inflamed conditions of the mucous membrane, hemorrhoids, piles, when rectal pain is in evidence, or in inflammatory diseases. Many pills sold for constipation contain aloes.

Aloes is also a stimulant to the uterus and vagina and has long been used as a household remedy to promote menstruation (amenorrhea). For this purpose, combine with an emmenagogue tonic and take in small doses.

A useful emmenagogue and cathartic is made by mixing 2 oz. each of powdered aloes and powdered myrrh and ½ oz. powdered ginger and filling #4 capsules.

In flatulence and constipation with uterine atony, take 1 or 2 capsules twice daily for a few days before the menstrual period.

From its special direction to the rectum, it has been found that powdered aloes in 1 gr. capsules every 3 hrs, will often clear out pin worms after a few doses.

A good hepatic and cathartic preparation is made by mixing 2 dr. FE aloes and 6 dr. FE dandelion into 4 oz. syrup of ginger.

With its other powers, aloes combines the property of slightly stimulating the stomach and is therefore, in minute doses, an excellent remedy in habitual constipation attended with torpor of the digestive organs (dyspepsia).

Given to nursing mothers, it causes purging in the suckling infant.

The fresh juice is used as an emollient (skin) for minor burns, blistered surfaces, sunburns, insect bites, etc. (Have you noticed the ads stressing aloes in skin creams recently put on the market?)

The medium dose of aloes is 10 gr.; but as a laxative, it will often operate in the quantity of 2 or 3 gr.; and when a decided impression is required, the dose may be augmented to 20 grs. In consequence of its excessively bitter taste, it is more conveniently administered in pill form. The dehydrated juice can also be used as a purgative.

Continued use of pills containing aloes will, in many cases, weaken the rectum.

The aloes mentioned in the Bible as a perfume for garments, beds, and burial is the gum of the eagle tree of India.

ASAFOETIDA (Ferula Asafoetida)

Asafoetide is a native of Persia and other countries of the East. It appears to have been known in the East from very early ages and, notwithstanding its repulsive odor, is at present much used in India and Persia as a condiment.

The oldest plants are most productive, and those under 4 years old are not considered worth cutting. The juice is collected and allowed to harden in the sun.

The odor is garlic-like, extremely fetid, and tenaceous; the taste is bitter, acrid, and long lasting. It is said 1 dr. of the fresh juice diffuses a more powerful odor through a closed room than 100# of the drug as usually kept in the stores.

Asafoetida softens by heat without melting and is difficult to pulverize. It yields all its virtues to alcohol and forms a clear tincture which becomes milky on the addition of water. When distilled whether with water or alcohol, it affords an essential oil upon which its odor and taste depend. It is ranked among the gum resins.

It is one of the best antispasmodics in hysteria, hypochondria, infantile convulsions and flatulent colic, convulsions of various kinds, spasms of the stomach and bowels unconnected with inflammation, and those numerous irregular and spasmodic nervous disorders which accompany derangement of the different organs or result from mere debility of the nervous system, restlessness, nervous irritability, insomnia, and has been most successfully used in spasmodic asthma, double vision, spermatorrhea, dysmenorrhea, and gastric irritation.

In congestion or inflammation of the brain, double vision, and meningitis, a useful antispasmodic is made as follows: mix together 1 dr. each powdered asafoetida, powdered valerian root, and 10 gr. powdered capsicum and fill into #4 capsules.

Its expectorant property is highly useful in spasmodic and pectoral affections such as whooping cough, asthma, croup, colds, bronchial troubles, infantile coughs and catarrhs complicated with disorders of the nervous system, debility, measles, catarrh, and in pulmonary consumption; in fact in all cases of diseases of the chest in which the lungs do not perform properly asafoetida may be taken to advantage.

In typhoid disease attended with excessive accumulation of air in the bowels or in the case of tympanitic abdomen, an enema may be of benefit. This may be found most convenient, also, in hysteric paroxysms and other kinds of convulsions.

Asafoetida may be combined with purgative medicines in constipation of the bowels with flatulence.

Dissolved and used as an enema in the evening, asafoetida will influence the bowels and the pelvic nerves if retained throughout the night. This is an excellent method to be used for the hysterical and the habitually nervous. The whole system will feel its effect, and by morning, the nerves will be thoroughly quieted. Mix ½ to 2 dr. in 4 oz. tepid water.

A syrup may be made by thoroughly mixing 1 oz. of the gum in boiling water, adding 2# sugar and enough water to fill 1 pt.

As asafoetida is not apt to affect the brain injuriously, it may be taken very freely when not contra-indicated by the existence of inflammatory action.

The tincture is official and is frequently used.

The medium dose is 10 gr. in pill or emulsion.

It seems impossible to cover either the taste or smell of this gum, and for this reason, it is frequently given in pill or capsule form.

BISTORT *(Polygonum Bistorta)*

This plant is a native of Europe and the north of Asia. Called "snakeweed" because it is supposed the leaves and the ROOTS have a powerful faculty to resist poison.

The ROOT is the official portion. The taste is astringent with no odor.

Bistort is one of the strongest astringents. It is used in gargles and in injections.

Useful in cases of diarrhea, dysentery, and cholera. If the bowels should be astringed, the following will be an excellent combination: infuse 1 oz. each crushed bistort root and raspberry leaves in 1½ pts. boiling water. Keep hot for ½ hr., strain the clear liquid on 1 t. composition powder, (see bayberry) and cover. Dose—adults 3 T. every ½ hr. until the purging is arrested. This will clear the canker from the mucous membrane of the alimentary canal, leaving it toned.

Bistort is a good wash for sore and ulcerated mouth and gums and is useful in internal and external hemorrhages and in enuresis. As an injection in leucorrhea, use the infusion.

May be employed in the form of decoction or powder. The dose of the powder is 20 or 30 gr., 3 or 4 times daily.

BUCHU *(Barosma Betulina)*

A small evergreen shrub, buchu is a native of the Cape of Good Hope. Called buchu in the language of the Hottentots by whom the leaves are highly esteemed for their odor and rubbed in the state of powder upon their greasy bodies. They have long used them in a variety of diseases. In fact, buchu is considered such a valuable plant that pedestrians are forbitten to pick it.

The odor is strong, diffusive, and somewhat aromatic; the taste bitterish and closely resembling mint. Water and alcohol extracts the virtues, which probably depends on the volatile oil contained in the leaves.

Buchu LEAVES are chiefly taken in complaints of the urinary organs, such as gravel, chronic catarrh of the bladder, morbid irritation of the bladder and urethra, disease of the prostate, the retention or incontinence of urine from a loss of tone in these parts, and has also been recommended in cutaneous affections.

A somewhat strong infusion taken cold is best to increase the flow of urine, while a warm infusion is gently diaphoretic and soothes the nerves. It will give valuable results in catarrh of the bladder, cystic catarrh, in congestion of the prostate with discharges and aching of the penis, in spermatorrhea, dropsy, and lingering leucorrhea.

In congestion of any of the pelvic organs, gleet, and mucous discharges in the urine, buchu will give good service.

Buchu readily eliminates the urates and relieves the system of uric acid through the urine. It has a very valuable influence in both acute and chronic rheumatism.

A good and somewhat stimulating diruetic is made as follows: Infuse in 1½ pts. boiling water 1 oz. buchu and ¼ oz. each juniper berries, cubebs, and uva ursi. Cover till cold, then strain and take 3 or 4 T. 3 times daily.

It will also exert quite an influence on the mucous membrane of the stomach. Is soothing to pelvic nerves and is used in an aching back and hips. In these conditions, it is useful to combine it with squaw vine (mitchella) or unicorn root. They will then assist in toning the generative organs.

If desired as a tonic, the leaves can be infused in brandy.

The infusion is a very acceptable remedy for aged people with urinary weakness.

For favorable results in leucorrhea, add an excess of Solomon's-seal. For a mildly stimulating nervine or diuretic add 4 parts tulip tree to 1 part buchu; for a relaxing nervine diuretic add 6 parts lady's slipper to 1 part buchu; and for an antispasmodic diuretic, add 5 parts blue cohosh to 1 part buchu.

From 20 to 30 gr. of the powder may be taken 2 or 3 times daily. The infusion is made by infusing 1 oz. leaves to 1 pt. boiling water which may be taken in doses of 1 or 2 fl. oz. The Fl. X may be used in doses of ½ to 1 dr. A tincture has also been used as a stimulant embrocation in local pains.

In purchasing, specify the short leaves, as they are considered superior to the long.

Buchu is best if NOT boiled.

CLOVES *(Caryophyllum Aromaticus)*

The clove tree was once confined to the Molucca Islands. Now the U.S. derives its chief supplies from Zanzibar.

The UNEXPANDED FLOWER BUDS are the part of the plant used, and are first gathered when the tree is 6 to 7 years old. It continues to bloom for almost 100 years. It is thought the full-blown flower and the fruit are destitute of aromatic properties.

The odor of cloves is strong and fragrant; their taste hot and pungent. The best cloves are large, heavy, brittle, and exude a small quantity of oil on being pressed or when scraped. Water extracts the odor of cloves with comparatively little of their taste. All their sensible properties are imparted to alcohol, and the tincture, when evaporated, leaves an excessively fiery extract.

Cloves are among the most stimulant of the aromatics. They are sometimes administered in substance or infusion to relieve nausea and vomiting, correct flatulence, and excite languid digestion; but their chief use is to modify the griping action and the unpleasant taste of other medicines. They enter as ingredients into several official preparations. Their dose in substance is from 5 to 10 grains.

In the vomiting of pregnancy, it is both safe and effectual. Combine powdered cloves and powdered white poplar bark in equal parts. Take about 20 grains, either as a powder or filled in capsules, upon the first appearance of vomiting.

The oil of cloves is a diffusive stimulant and is often rubbed on the gum to relieve toothache and frequently is used as a specific for offensive breath.

Domestically cloves are used as a spice and flavoring. Its fragrance makes it one of the principal ingredients in sachets, pomanders, pot pourris, cosmetics, and soaps.

Clove pomanders were once very popular. They were used to perfume and to protect clothing and linens from moths.

EUROPEAN COLUMBO *(Cocculus Palamatus)*

This climbing plant is a native of and grows wild in Mozambique, Africa. The American columbo is the root of the *Frasera Carolinesis*, which is sometimes used as a substitute.

It is claimed the name columbo derives from the city of Columbo in Ceylon, from which the herb was exported, but it is also believed a more probable derivation is from the word "calumb," which is said to be the Mozambique name for the root. Natives call it "kalumb."

Columbo is among the most useful and valuable of the tonics.

The virtues of the ROOT are extracted by boiling water and by alcohol. The ROOT is brittle and easily pulverized but spoils by keeping after having been reduced to powder. It is best to powder as it is required for use.

Columbo influences chiefly the mucous membrane of the alvine tract. It invigorates the stomach, improves the appetite, and assists digestion and assimilation.

Being without astringency, it is generally acceptable to the stomach and is an excellent remedy in simple dyspepsia and those states of debility attending convalescence from acute disorders, especially of the alimentary canal. Hence it is often prescribed in the declining stages of remittent fever, dysentery, diarrhea, cholera morbus, and cholera infantum. The absence of irritating properties renders it also an appropriate tonic in hectic fever of phthisis and its kindred affections. It is frequently combined with other tonics, with aromatics and mild cathartics, and with antacids.

The following is most effective in a disposition to the accumulation of flatus in the bowels: infuse ½ oz. each powdered columbo and powdered ginger and 1 dr. senna in 1 pt. boiling water. Cover till cold and take in dose of 1 wine-glassful 3 times daily.

Columbo is much used by the natives of Mozambique and the neighboring parts of Africa in dysentery and other diseases. An astringent could be added. Columbo, by combining with other remedies, may be made to influence any particular part of the mucous membrane.

As a tonic it may be substituted for Peruvian bark. It is soothing to the mucous membrane, will not excite nausea, and is of excellent service in allaying the vomiting of pregnancy. It is a much milder tonic than gentian; and is valuable in all cases of dyspepsia, weak and irritated conditions of the stomach, and can be used safely with good effect both before and after confinement.

In convalescence from fevers, where the mucous membrane of the alvine tract is in an irritated condition, it is a good remedy. In pulmonary consumption, it is a most useful tonic, having a slightly demulcent property and having no stimulating effect upon the bowels. It has no tendency to purge and, because of this, is often used in combination with other pulmonary remedies.

The following is a formula used for weak and impaired digestion: boil in 1 qt. water 1 oz. each columbo root, white poplar bark and raspberry leaves, and ½ oz. horehound for 15 min. Strain while hot on ½ t. cayenne. Dose ½ wine-glassful 3 or 4 times daily.

Columbo is most commonly used in infusion. The dose of the powder is from 10 to 30 grains and may be repeated 3 or 4 times daily. It is frequently combined with powdered ginger.

CUBEBS *(Piper Cubebs)*

Cubebs are native to Java where it grows luxuriantly in the woods and which furnishes much of the cubebs for commerce. They are not cultivated. The fruits or berries are called tailed pepper and also Java pepper after the port from which they were originally shipped.

The odor of the berry is agreeably aromatic; the taste warm, bitterish, and camphorous, leaving in the mouth a peculiar sensation of coolness, like that produced by the oil of peppermint. The unripe FRUIT is used.

Cubebs gradually deteriorate by age, and in the state of powder become weaker, in consequence of the escape of some active volatile ingredient. They should always be kept whole and pulverized at the time of using them.

Cubebs are gently stimulant, influencing the mucous membrane, especially the urinary organs. In hot infusion, they usually excite the circulation, increase the heat of the body, and promote the flow of urine, to which they impart a peculiar odor. They are said to give rise to a sense of coolness in the rectum during the passage of the feces.

There is no evidence that they were known to the ancients. They were probably first brought into Europe by the Arabians. They were brought into notice as a remedy in gonorrhea and have

135

been found very efficient in this complaint. This application of cubebs was derived from India, where they have long been used in gonorrhea, gleet, seminal weakness, and leucorrhea. The following is excellent: Simmer 1 oz. white pond lily and ½ oz. American mandrake in 1 quart water for 15 min., then pour on 1 oz. cubebs. Cover till cold. Strain and take 2 to 4 T., 3 or 4 times daily. It is a grateful stomachic and carminative in disorders of the digestive organs.

They will be found most safe and effectual in cases of inflammation of the mucous membrane of the urethra and are best taken in the form of powder of which the dose is 1 to 3 drachms., repeated 3 or 4 times daily.

They will manifest quite an influence in the mucous membrane in cleaning up discharges of the urinary organs, and in scalding urine they will be found useful. The berries may be crushed and ½ t. taken in ½ C. cold water, 3 times daily.

Their use is NOT best in ACUTE inflammatory conditions, but excellent in chronic conditions as gleet and cystic catarrh.

In cystic and nephritic congestions and chronic inflammatory conditions, cubebs are sometimes combined with copaiba.

In nasal congestion, cubeb berries can be added to any tobacco mixture used for smoking.

The oil may be used in doses of 3 to 10 drops in sugar or in capsule form.

EUROPEAN OR YELLOW GENTIAN (*Gentiana Lutea*)

This plant grows among the Appenines, the Alps, the Pyrenees, and in other mountainous or elevated regions of Europe. It is now imported from Germany.

It has been used as a medicine by the ancients, and it is said to have derived its name from Gentius, a King of Illyria.

A fermented and distilled infusion is much relished as a liquor by the Swiss and the Tyrolese.

The ROOT is the only part used in medicine. The taste is slightly sweetish and intensely bitter without being nauseous. The odor is feeble but decided and peculiar. The powder is of a yellowish color. Water and alcohol extract its taste and medical virtues.

Gentian is one of our finest tonics. It is an old favorite for promoting the appetite, tones the powers of digestion, moderately increases the temperature of the body, stimulates the circulation, and acts, in fact, as a general strengthener of the system. Doses should be reasonably small.

Many of the complex preparations handed down from the Greeks and the Arabians contain it among their ingredients, and it enters into most of the stomachic combinations employed in modern practice. It may be used in all cases of disease dependent on pure debility of the digestive organs or requiring a general tonic impression; dyspepsia, gout, amenorrhea, hysteria, scrofula, intermittent fever, diarrhea, worms, are among the many forms of diseases in which it will prove useful, but it is the conditions of the stomach and of the system generally which must be taken into consideration, and there is scarcely a single complaint in which it cannot be used advantageously. Its powder has been applied externally to malignant and sloughing ulcers.

It is taken, usually, in the form of infusion of 1 T to a wineglassful, 3 times daily, or the tincture of 1 or 2 t. The dose of the powder is from 10 to 40 grains.

In languid conditions and general debility, it is one of the best tonics. Its effect upon the liver is that of a cholagogue, rather than to influence the secretion of bile. It is of extreme value in jaundice and bilious conditions and is much used in this disease.

Gentian influences the portal (venous) circulation somewhat similar to golden seal.

A pleasant and mildly stimulating tonic can be made as follows: 1 oz. gentian, 2 oz. each coriander seed and orange peel and ¼ oz. cinnamon. Make an infusion, using 1 oz. to 1 pt. boiling water. Dose from 2 to 3 T., 3 or 4 times daily.

In general use, it is best combined with an aromatic.

An excellent tonic for a weak stomach with poor digestion is made as follows: 1 dr. FE gentian and 4 oz. syr. ginger. Take just before meals.

Gentian is considered a most useful vegetable tonic; and one of the best strengtheners of the human system. It should always be carried in one's purse so as to be ready to be used upon all occasions; steeped in wine and drunk, it refreshes the exhausted.

A simple way to obtain the benefits of gentian is to purchase some angostura aromatic bitters. The label will read that it contains gentian and also the directions for using. Angostura bitters is a nervine tonic, and when added to a glass of milk, plus some powdered milk for added calcium, with an egg and a little sugar, it will make a beneficial and pleasant drink.

GINGER *(Zingiberis Officinale)*

The Jamaica ginger is considered the best, although some ginger is now being cultivated in Florida. This is not to be confused with the wild ginger *(Asarum Canadense)*, also known as the Canada snakeroot.

A native of Hindustan, ginger is one of the most ancient of spices. It was brought to the New World by the Spaniards early in the 16th century. The unpeeled are sold as black or green ginger, and the peeled is sold as the white or Jamaica ginger. Our supply usually comes from Jamaica.

The ROOT is the portion in which the medicinal virtues reside. This is dug up when 1 yr. old.

The odor is aromatic and penetrating, the taste is spicy, pungent, hot, and biting. These properties gradually diminish as the root is exposed. Their virtues are extracted by water and alcohol.

In cooking and for teas, the powdered form of ginger is most used. Gingerbread, gingersnaps, ginger ale, wine, and tea are probably the most popular, and surely pumpkin pie would never be the same without it. Crystalized ginger (young and tender roots boiled in syrup) is considered a fine confection. This is occasionally imported from the East and West Indies.

It is often taken for dyspepsia, flatulent colic, and in the feeble state of the alimentary canal attendant upon atonic gout. Added to bitter infusions and tonic powders, ginger warms the stomach.

It is an excellent remedy in typhoid and other fevers and all the eruptive diseases, especially with fever, and in bronchitis, pneumonia, and angina.

It us useful in flatulence, internal congestions, spasms, recent colds, chills, dysentery, and diarrhea, and helps a sluggish circulation. Dose of 10 to 20 gr. in warm water, sweetened.

To relieve congested menstrual flow, drink hot 1 t. of the powder in 1 C. boiling water, sweeten, cover, allow to stand a few minutes.

Chewing a little ginger root will stimulate the salivary gland producing a copious flow of saliva. This is useful in paralysis of the tongue and fauces, relaxation of the uvula, sore throat, flatulence, and colic, and helpful in hemorrhage of the lungs.

Used with cathartics, it will prevent nausea and griping.

Ginger is much more diffusive than capsicum and can be used as a substitute.

If a mild laxative is desired, the following will be useful; place about 20 senna leaves in a cup, ¼ t. powdered ginger, a slice of lemon, and 1 t. sugar. Pour on ⅓ C. boiling water, cover, and allow to stand until it can be drunk conveniently. Take all in one dose, the liquid only. This, taken warm, is a very pleasant drink, and no griping will result.

An excellent cordial for chills and colds is made by adding ginger to whiskey according to taste. Let stand 2 weeks, strain.

1 part ginger and 4 parts pleurisy root forms an excellent diaphoretic.

With lobelia, ginger increases its anti-spasmodic power.

The tincture may be used for all the same purposes; dose 5 to 20 min.

The infusion may be prepared by adding ½ oz. of powdered or bruised root to 1 pt. boiling water and taken in doses of 1 or 2 fl. oz.

MISTLETOE *(Viscum Album)*

The mistletoe of the U.S. is the *phorandendron flavenscens,* the Oklahoma state flower.

Mistletoe is a true vegetable parasite which sends suckers penetrating through the bark of the host tree, thus obtaining nourishment from it.

In the Dark Ages, superstition surrounded this plant. It was considered sacred because of a belief that mistletoe did not grow from seeds but from bird droppings, because it grew only high in the trees and never on the ground.

People hung it around their necks and from the ceilings of their homes to repel witchcraft and ward off evil spirits. Mistletoe is still used today in many homes at Christmastime.

The Saxons, at the commencement of the New Year, distributed mistletoe plants among the people as a sacred relic; it was deemed a panacea against every disease and remedy for poisons.

Birds eat the fruit.

Mistletoe also produces a substance known as bird-lime which is excessively sticky and is used on fly-papers.

The WHOLE PLANT is used, leaves, berries, and twigs. It should be gathered when the berries are ripe and, after drying, kept in air-tight containers.

Its principal use is as a nervine.

Mistletoe is considered a specific in chorea. Its nervine and tonic properties make it of great value in epilepsy, convulsions, hysteria, delirium, nervous debility, or any trouble caused by weakness or disordered state of the nervous system; it quiets the nerves, will lessen cerebral excitement, and will favorably influence febrile conditions. Make a decoction using 1 oz. herb to 1 pt. water and take from 1 to 3 T. (according to age) every 1, 2, or 3 hours. There will be no unpleasant reaction as with bromides.

A good remedy for nervous troubles is made by simmering ½ oz. of each mistletoe, valerian rt., and vervain herb in 1½ pts. water for 10 min. Strain and take 2 T. 3 times daily.

If the digestive organs are weak, add a little cayenne.

During parturition, when pains are light, it produces prompt uterine contractions, will anticipate hemorrhage, and will assist in the expulsion of the placenta, when retained. In all uterine hemorrhages, it is useful.

Its antispasmodic properties will be useful in the relief of asthma, epilepsy, and other spasmodic conditions.

MYRRH *(Balsamodendron Myrrha)*

Genesis 37:25 (BC 1729)—(Spice Commerce)—"A company of Ishmaelites came from Gilead, with their camels, bearing spicery and balm and MYRRH going to carry it down to Egypt." Exodus 30:23, 24, 25, 30, 31 (BC 1491)—(The Holy anointing oil)—"The Lord spake unto Moses, saying: Take thou unto thee principal spices; of pure MYRRH 500 shekels and of sweet cinnamon ½ as much and of sweet calamus 250 shekels and of cassia 250 shekels, after the shekel of the sanctuary and of olive oil an hin; and thou shalt make it an oil of holy ointment."

Matt. 2:11—(Birth of Christ and visit of the wise men)—"They presented Him gifts; gold, frankincense, and MYRRH."

Mark 15:23 (A.D. 33)—(At crucifixion of Christ)—"And they gave Him to drink wine mingled with MYRRH."

John 19:39, 40—(A.D. 33)—(The death and burial of Jesus)—"And there came also Nicodemus, which at first came to Jesus by night, and brought a mixture of MYRRH and Aloes, about 100# weight. They took the body of Jesus and wound it in linen clothes with the spices."

According to an ancient legend, the gum resin of myrrh is the bitter tears of Myrrha whom the Gods turned into the myrrh shrub to protect her from her drunken father. He was Theias, the King of Assyria.

Myrrh has been used in medicines and incense from the earliest periods of history. It grows in Arabia, Abyssinia, and Somaliland.

It is one of the ingredients in the incense Moses fixed for the Jewish ceremonial rites and was used as a medicine by the ancients.

There are 2 varieties on the market; the India and the Turkey myrrh. The Turkey myrrh generally excels in quality.

The JUICE exudes spontaneously and CONCRETES upon the bark. No cut is necessary. Alcohol and water severally extract the whole of its odor and taste. It is best to powder it first, when using in decoction or infusion.

This GUM is a slow, mild, stimulating, antiseptic tonic with some tendency to the lungs and to the uterus. Hence it is employed as an expectorant and emmenagogue in debilitated states of the system, in the absence of febrile excitement or acute inflammation. The complaints for which it is usually taken, are chronic catarrh, phthisis pulmonalis, humoral asthma, and other pectoral affections in which secretion of mucus is abundant but not easily expectorated, chlorosis, amenorrhea, and the various affections connected with this state of the uterine function. In amenorrhea, it is frequently combined with aloes.

The infusion is sometimes taken but the X has been recommended as being the mildest. The tincture is used chiefly as an external application.

The tincture forms a fine wash for sores, spongy and inflamed gums, the aphthous sore mouth of children, and various kinds of unhealthy ulcers. A little taken internally will help in removing bad breath. In using the tincture as a mouth wash or gargle, mix 1 t. with 2 T. tepid water. It can, of course, be made stronger or weaker, if desired. As a gargle in diphtheria, inflammatory sore or relaxed throat, thrush, bad legs, ulceration of the tongue, mouth, and throat. Sprayed into the mouth and down the throats of infants in these conditions, it is a fine remedy.

The powdered gum is a good application for sores and ulcers and is also useful to apply to the umbilicus of the infant after removing the cord. It will assist the healing process, removing foul odors and arresting putrefaction.

2 to 5 drops of the FE will be found useful to relieve fermentation in atonic indigestion and nausea incident to pregnancy.

It will diminish mucous discharges and is therefore useful in some chest affections as cough, asthma, and tuberculosis in combination with other remedies. It can be used in substance, fluid X, tincture, or infusion. In taking powder, 2 to 5 gr. will be a sufficient dose.

When taken in a hot infusion, myrrh stimulates the circulation and assists a flow of blood toward the capillaries and will give a sense of pleasant warmth to the stomach.

Myrrh tends to prevent septic conditions, purifies the blood current and rapidly increases the white blood corpuscles.

An antiseptic, diffusive tonic for the circulation and nervous system is made as follows: mix 4 dr. ea. FE myrrh and FE lady's slipper, 20 dr. FE prickly ash into 4 oz. syr. of ginger.

Because of its astringent, healing tonic and stimulating properties, myrrh is an excellent tooth powder.

The following is a valuable antiseptic: mix 4 oz. pulverized myrrh and 2 Dr. pulverized cayenne into 1 oz. simple syrup.

A few drops in water taken before an anasthesia will sustain the heart, steady the nerves, and cause a fuller and better pulse.

One drop in water, repeated as needed, is an excellent parturient. It equalizes the circulation, sustains the contractions, relieves irritability, and anticipates flooding. Do not take any other stimulant unless needed.

In shock from injury, there is nothing better.

An old herbalist claims that myrrh will take away the wrinkles that come of age and make the face smooth and youthful; he calls it "liquor of myrrh." Here is his recipe: boil eggs hard;

take out the yolks and fill centers with powdered myrrh; put in a glass and set in a wine-cellar or moist place; wash the face with the liquor. Use before bedtime for 8 consecutive days.

BLACK PEPPER *(Piper Nigrum)*

Black pepper vines grow in the East Indies, Java, and Sumatra. We are told that the best pepper grows in Malabar but that the U.S. derives their chief supply from Sumatra and Java. They bear fruit only after 3 or 4 years.

The black and white peppers are the FRUIT of the piper nigrum.

For black pepper, the BERRIES are gathered before they are fully ripe, and upon being dried in the sun, become black and wrinkled.

For the white pepper, the BERRIES from the same plant, are gathered when fully ripe, soaked in water until the external coat peels off, and then dried in the sun. The white is less pungent than the black, however the black is the more popular.

The use of pepper is centuries old. It was demanded in payment of taxes by the Greeks before the time of Christ. It was considered more valuable than gold and silver, being more difficult to secure. Early in the 10th century, English landlords taxed their tenants 1# pepper annually.

Pepper became so valuable and important that, in 1937, the N. Y. Pepper Exchange was organized.

From the time of Hippocrates, it has been employed as a condiment and as a medicine. Its culinary uses are too well-known to require explanation.

The dried, black BERRIES have an aromatic smell and a hot pungent and most fiery taste. They yield their virtues partially to water and entirely to alcohol.

Black pepper is an active stimulant and will assist in producing perspiration. It has some reputation as a gastro-intestinal stimulant to excite the languid stomach, assist digestion, and correct flatulence. It may be used as a substitute for cayenne.

It is capable of producing general arterial excitement. In hot infusion, it stimulates the circulation and tends to flow toward the surface. It assists in keeping up the temperature of the body and prevents exhaustion. Useful in congestive chills.

In the past, it was used for intermittents, however the bark was considered superior and the alcoholic X of pepper more so. In those cases of intermittents in which the stomach is not duly susceptible to the action of quinine, as in some instances of alcoholics, pepper may be found to be a useful adjuvant to the more powerful febrifuge.

The dose of pepper is from 5 to 20 grains. It may be taken in berry or powder, but is more energetic in powder form. The oil may be triturated on sugar.

Black pepper, red pepper, cayenne, and ginger maintains heat of the body longer than any other remedy. Black pepper is much used as a corrective of coldness and flatulence of a vegetable diet and is much adapted to our warm climate.

The *New England Homestead* once wrote: "as a moth repellent, sprinkle black pepper liberally among blankets and woolens, into suits and coat pockets before storing for the summer. Moths seem to hate it, and it is easily brushed, shaken, and aired out."

PERUVIAN BARK *(Cinchona)*

It has been written that genuine cinchona trees grow wild in So. America, principally in the region of Bogota, Peru, but some are now cultivated in Europe. Many varieties have been found, even one in Georgia and So. Carolina, which was aptly called *Cinchona Caroliniana*.

Although discovery has been ascribed to the Jesuits, the natives of Peru knew the febrifuge power of cinchona long before the civilized world became acquainted with it.

The Jesuits were sent to Peru as missionaries. It was during this period that tertain ague was a prevalent disorder. They administered an infusion of cinchona and soon ascertained its extraordinary powers.

The Countess of Chinchon, wife of the Spanish Viceroy of Peru, after being cured of fever with this bark, returned to Spain in 1640 and introduced the remedy into Europe. It was then sold by the Jesuits under the name of "Jesuit's powder," a name it long retained.

In France it was employed, with great success, in the treatment of intermittents under the name of "English powder." During this period, the actual remedy was held a secret. In 1679 the secret preparation was sold to Louis XIV, by whom it was divulged.

It is from the BARK of the cinchona tree that quinine is derived. Taking quinine to excess has often resulted in buzzing in the ears and deafness. Quinine should only be taken under the supervision of a physician.

In using the BARK, however, in its natural state, it is most useful.

The most popular types of Cinchona are as follows:

Cinchona Calisaya is the yellow bark.

Cinchona Officinalis is the pale bark.

Cinchona Succirrubra is the red bark.

The red and pale varieties are considered more astringent, but it is claimed that the yellow furnishes the most quinine in proportion to bulk.

In the treatment of intermittents, either the red or the yellow bark is decidedly preferable to the pale. The red is usually considered the most powerful. The pale is considered superior as a tonic.

All of these varieties are stimulating nervines.

Cinchona is considered as ranking at the very head of the tonics. But, besides the mere excitation of the ordinary functions of health, it produces other effects upon the system which must be considered peculiar and wholly independent of its mere tonic operation. The power by which, when administered in the intervals between the paroxysms of intermittent disorders, it breaks the chain of morbid association and interrupts the progress of the disease, is something more than what is usually understood by the tonic property; for no other substance belonging to the class, however powerful or permanent the excitement which it produces, exhibits a control over intermittents at all comparable to that of cinchona. From the possession both of the tonic, and of the anti-intermittent property, the bark is capable of being usefully applied in the treatment of a great number of diseases.

It is in the treating of intermittent diseases that the bark displays its most extraordinary powers. It was originally introduced to notice as a remedy in fever and ague, and the reputation which it acquired at any early period, it has ever since retained. Very few cases of this disease will be found to resist the judicious use of the bark or some of its preparations.

Early employment in SMALL doses (1 or 2 oz.) is recommended, preferably diffused in water or some aromatic infusion.

Experience has proven that its efficacy in the intermittents is often greatly promoted by mixing with powdered Virginia snake root.

The medium dose of bark as taken in intermittents is 1 drachm., to be repeated more or less according to circumstances. When taken as a tonic in chronic complaints, the dose is usually smaller, from 10 to 30 grains, being sufficient to commence.

Cinchona includes in its range of influence, the entire nervous system; the sympathetic, the cerebral, spinal, and the peripheral as well as the central nerves.

Its tonic properties will be found effective in incontinence of urine.

For an excellent general tonic, boil 1 qt. of water with the following: ½ oz. each Peruvian bark, gentian root, orange peel, columbo root, and liqorice and about ⅛ t. cayenne for 15 min. Cool, strain, and take ½ C. ev. 3 hrs. during the day.

Spasmodic conditions arising from weakness may be quieted by cinchona.

Cinchona is employed with benefit in all morbid conditions of the system providing the stomach, liver, bowels, and circulation are functioning properly. If necessary, add anti-bilious or physic remedies to the cinchona dose.

Cinchona is also useful in low or typhoid fever, either with or minus inflammation or in the suppurative or gangrenous stage, in typhus gravior, malignant scarlatina, measles, and smallpox, in carbuncle and gangrenous erysipelis, and in all cases in which the system is exhausted under large purulent discharges.

As a tonic, the bark is advantageously employed in chronic diseases connected with debility; as for example, in scrofula, dropsy, passive hemorrhages, certain forms of dyspepsia, obstinate cutaneous affections, amenorrhea, chorea, hysteria; in fact, whenever a strengthening influence is desired. Particularly those of a neuralgic character, migraine and violent pains in the eye, face, and other parts of the body, occurring periodically, are often almost immediately relieved by the use of the bark.

When large doses are deemed necessary, fill the ears with lady's slipper and lobelia repeating at intervals as needed. It prevents the presence of the extreme tension upon the auditory nerves.

The simple infusion is made steeping 1 t. bark in 1 C. boiling water for ½ hr. Drink 1 C. during the day.

Peruvian bark can be freely used as a mouth wash and gargle.

WOOD OR GARLIC SAGE *(Teucrium Scorodonia)*

This plant grows wild in Great Britain. Its taste is bitter and its odor is slightly aromatic.

As an alterative and tonic, it is very healing, preventing mortification or gangrene. Used in diseases of the blood and skin troubles and valuable as a restorer after an acute attack of rheumatism or gout. It will freely influence the bladder and increase the flow of urine when combined with comfrey and ragwort. It is considered equal to gentian as a stimulant to the appetite.

Combine with chickweed in equal parts when used as a poultice in indolent ulcers, boils, and swellings.

May also be used as an infusion in obstructed menstruation, colds, fevers, and inflammation. Take wine-glassful doses of warm infusion made of 1 oz. in 1 pint boiling water.

SANICLE also called Wood Sanicle *(Sanicula Europea)*

An old Italian proverb says: "He who hath self-heal and sanicle needs no other physician."

Wood sanicle is a native of England. The taste is bitter, astringent, and subsequently acrid with no odor.

It is an extremely useful remedy and extensively used in blood disorders. It is most effectual in cleansing the system of morbid secretions, thereby leaving the blood stream in a much better condition.

It is considered a specific for scurvy and excellent in scrofulous and catarrh conditions. Also excellent for ulcers in the mouth and throat, for which drink and gargle freely a decoction of 1 oz. to 1 pt. Use this also as a gargle in sore throat, quinsy, and to cleanse the throat of mucus.

In external ulcers and running sores, a wash will be useful.

It is also useful in leucorrhea, diarrhea and dysentery, and in inflammation of the bronchi and pulmonary troubles. This herb alone or combined with a little ginger, sweetened and taken in a strong decoction at the rate of 1 pint a day is used with splendid results in pulmonary consumption.

In ulceration of the lungs and stomach, use the following: simmer 1 qt. water with 1 oz. sanicle and ½ oz. each marshmallow root and mullein herb for 5 min. Cover and allow to stand until warm. Strain and take from 4 to 8 T. every 3 hrs.

A hot infusion may be used to advantage in colds with fever, whether of the head or the respiratory organs, and in the fever stage of the eruptive disease, especially in measles.

In scald head, tetters, and other cases of rashes, either the infusion or the decoction used externally is one of the most effective remedies.

The infusion made of 1 oz. of the ROOT or herb to 1 pt. boiling water is taken in wine-glassful doses.

The American sanicle is *Sanicula Marilandica*.

SANTONICA *(Artimisia Santonica)*

Originating in Russia, santonica is called "Levant wormseed" in Europe.

The seeds or unexpanded flower buds are used. It has a very strong aromatic odor and a very bitter, disagreeable taste. It contains a volatile oil in which its virtues reside.

From early times, santonica has been used as a remedy for worms. The old Arabic doctor of medicine used it. It can be used for tape, round, or seat worms, especially for round or stomach worms. There seems to be a difference of opinion among herbalists as to which worms santonica would prove effective.

The vermifuge action is due to the presence of santonine in the flowerheads. When extracted, it becomes a white crystal, almost tasteless, which is largely prescribed for children with worms. A dose of from 1 to 2 grains in 1 spoonful of water, given night and morning for 3 days and, if needed, followed by a cathartic, will frequently bring away the worms as a mass of mucus. Some take a cathartic in the morning after a dose of santonine at night, while others require no cathartic. It is a strong gastric tonic.

An injection made as follows is generally effective in a few days for pin worms: make a solution of 3 or 4 grains of santonine in water and inject once or twice daily.

Enuresis is sometimes caused by stomach or pin worms. Santonine will relieve this condition.

Santonine, in a few hours, might color the urine quite yellow.

148

Levant wormseed must not be confused with the proper (U.S.) wormseed *(Chenopodium Anthelminticum)*.

JAMAICA SARSAPARILLA *(Smilax Officinalis)*

The native American sarsaparilla is called *Smilax Sarsaparilla*. It is claimed it does not possess the same properties as the imported.

The name "sarsaparilla" is expressive of the character of the plant, being derived from two Spanish words which signify a small thorny vine. It is called zarzaparilla by the natives.

The Jamaica or red sarsaparilla is most commonly used in the U.S. and is considered superior to any of the other kinds. It is said to derive that name from the Island of Jamaica, which is the channel of its exportation from Honduras to Europe. The reddish color of its epidermis is its chief peculiarity.

Sarsaparilla, in its ordinary state, is nearly or quite inodorous, but in decoction it acquires a decided and peculiar smell. To the taste, it is mucilaginous and very slightly bitter and when chewed for some time produces a disagreeable acrid impression which remains long in the mouth and fauces. The ROOT is efficient in proportion as it possesses this acrimony. The bark is more powerful than the interior portions.

The virtues of the ROOT are communicated to water, cold or hot, but are impaired by long boiling. They are also extracted by diluted alcohol.

It is an excellent blood purifier, but is rarely taken alone. It is useful in scrofulous cases, rheumatism and chronic rheumatism, gout, skin eruptions.

In hot infusion, it gives an outward circulation of the blood.

A beer made by fermenting an infusion with molasses is said to be a popular remedy in So. America. It is made as follows: 2# bruised sarsaparilla, powdered bark of guaiacum 8 oz., raspings of guaiac wood, anise seed and licorice root of each 4 oz., mezereon (bark of root) 2 oz., molasses 2# and 1 dz. bruised cloves. Pour on these ingredients 4 gal. boiling water and shake 3 times daily. When fermentation has well begun, it is fit for use. May be taken in a dose of a small tumblerful 2 or 3 times daily. The bark of guaiacum may be omitted without materially affecting the virtues of the preparation.

A good compound decoction of sarsaparilla is made as follows:

Jamaica sarsaparilla 4 oz., burdock rt. 1 oz., guaiacum chips 1 oz., Clivers 1 oz., fumitory 1 oz., licorice rt. 1 oz. Pour on 3½ qts. water and simmer down to 2 qts. Strain and take ½ teacupful 3 or 4 times daily before meals. This is a good blood purifier.

For rheumatism, add to the above, when finished and cold, tincture prickly ash 1 oz. and tinct. queen's delight ½ oz. Some add to each pint, ½ dr. iodide of potassium.

Sarsaparilla may be taken in powder in dose of ½ dr. or a dr. 3 or 4 times daily, but it is more conveniently administered in the form of infusion, decoction, syrup, and FE.

SENNA (Cassia Acutifolia)

Senna grows wild in great abundance on the Mediterranean coast of Africa, in the vicinity of Tripoli. It is known commercially as "Tripoli senna," receiving the name Tripoli from the place of export.

Senna was first used as a medicine by the Arabians. It was noticed in their writings as early as the 9th century, and the name itself is Arabic.

The odor is faint and sickly; the taste is slightly bitter, sweetish, and nauseous. Water and alcohol extract its active principle.

The ROOTS, LEAVES, and PODS are a prompt, stimulating cathartic, action being brought about in from 2 to 5 hours. While it does not produce the watery evacuations produced by epsom salts, it thoroughly influences peristaltic action. The addition of a little ginger, cloves, coriander seeds, or peppermint will prevent griping in the bowels. Small doses may be continued for some time without tiring the system. It is a prompt, efficient, and safe purgative, especially for fevers and febrile complaints and other cases in which a decided but not violent impression is desired.

An excellent anti-bilious physic is prepared as follows: all in powder, senna 2 oz., jalap 4 oz., ginger ¼ oz. Mix. May be taken in a little water, either with or without sugar, or in capsule form or in a little jam. If a speedy action is desired, take a fairly large dose and rest. Good alvine action will result in from 2 to 3 hrs., relieving engorgement of the liver and gall ducts. Small doses taken every 3 hrs. will influence the liver more than the alvine canal.

It stimulates and cleanses the alvine mucous membrane. It is useful in jaundice where the overflow is not from gallstones.

Eruptive diseases will follow a less virulent course and a more favorable termination if the bowels are thoroughly cleansed at the beginning.

In chronic or acute constipation, first take a dose sufficient to procure a complete evacuation, then take smaller doses, gradually decreasing the frequency and quantity. In the meantime, strive for habitual regularity. Can be given in suitable doses to infants.

The anti-bilious physic has been used in the treatment of remittents and intermittents with much success. It will also anticipate and prevent a chill and will frequently do it more permanently than quinine. It will prevent the necessity of taking so much quinine as would otherwise be required.

It is excellent to use after an anthelmintic.

For hemorrhoids, the compound should be taken in small doses every 3 hours.

The following can be used if a simple infusion is not strong enough; all in powder, equal parts of senna, mandrake, and cloves. Mix and take 1 or 2 dr. in honey, syrup, or jam, or it may be taken in capsules.

The senna PODS are an old-time remedy. Place 8 or 10 pods in a glass of lukewarm water and allow to soak about 12 hrs. Drink the whole liquid at night before retiring. A little ginger could be added.

A good preparation for children is made as follows: equal parts of senna, pennyroyal, and raspberry leaves. Infuse and give as strong and as frequently as required.

The following has been used with most satisfactory results for many years in cases of biliousness and constipation: about 25 rubbed senna leaves (1 t.), powdered ginger ¼ t., sugar 1 t., a slice of lemon. Pour on 1 C. boiling water. Cover and drink the whole while warm, leaving the powder, of course. This makes a very pleasant drink and can be given to children as ginger wine.

When combined with tonics, the effects of senna will be more powerful.

A good infusion is made of 2 oz. senna leaves, 1 dr. ginger in 1 pt. boiling water. Let stand 1 hr. Strain through muslin and take in wine-glassful doses.

The American senna is the *Cassia Marilandica*. It is often substituted for the European senna, but is less active, a ⅓ larger dose must be used to obtain the same results.

DISEASES

Part II

ABDOMEN—The visceral cavity
>*see* Alvine Canal, Rupture, Peritonitis
Chronic engorgement of the viscera—Elecampane
Irritated and inflamed—Wild Yam, Roman Chamomile
Pain—Lady's Slipper
Tympantic (Inflammation)—Asafoetida
Dropsy—Dandelion

ABSCESSES (Imposthumes)—Cavities containing pus
>*see* Boils, Carbuncles
Breast (Mammary)—*see* Blood purifiers
Painful chronic—Mullein, Sassafras
Useful—Carrot, Red Elm, Figwort, Ground Ivy, Linseed, Marshmallow, Sassafras
Anus Fistula—Yarrow

ACID—Sour conditions
>*see* Charcoal, Hiccough
To neutralize stomach acids, which often lead to ulcers—drink half glass whole milk or half glass of half milk and half cream every hour, except at meal time.
Specific in sour stomach and regurgitation of food—Black Horehound

ACNE—*see* Blood impurities

ADENOIDS—Small spongy growth in the roof of the throat. If enlarged, because of unhealthy conditions, it can prevent passage of air from the inner ear to the throat, causing earache and deafness.
Dry up and clean out mucus—Bayberry

AGUE—Intermittent malarial fever with periodic chill
>*see* fevers, chills

AIR PURIFICATION—planting of sunflowers and eucalyptus freely in malarious regions is supposed to do away with the danger of malaria. It is considered also very effective if planted close to the house.
Chronic—Boneset cannot be excelled
Tertian—Peruvian Bark
Useful—Boneset, Peruvian Bark, Sunflower Leaves, Blessed Thistle

155

ALBUMINURIA—Albumin in the urine is one of the first symptoms of the existence of Bright's disease.
    see Bright's Disease, Kidneys, Urine
  Of great value—False Unicorn

ALCOHOLIC—One suffering the morbid effects of excessive use of alcoholic beverages
  Delirium—Hops
  Dilated blood vessels reduced—Cayenne
  Dispel stupor and drowsiness—Coffee, Kola
  To make a man sober—eat Cabbage
  Useful—Black Pepper

ALIMENTARY CANAL—Food passage from mouth to anus
    see Flatulent, intestinal
  Atonic—Juniper
  Canker—Bistort
  Enfeebled—Eur Columbo, Ginger
  Irritated in infants—Rhubarb
  Influence secretions throughout whole of canal—Yarrow

ALVINE CANAL—Abdomen (stomach and bowels)
    see Colitis, Intestinal, Mucous Membrane
  Languid and sluggish—Serpentaria
  Scrofula—Poke
  Stimulates—Horseradish
  Tonic—Balmony, Amer & Eur Columbo, Cranesbill, Butternut
  Useful—Butternut, Linseed, Maidenhair, Senna

AMENORRHEA—Absence of or suppressed menses
    see Menstruation
  Congestion or obstruction—Motherwort, G. Rue
  Hysteria—Peppermint
  Increases or promotes—Aloes, Ro. Chamomile, Black Cohosh, Elecampane, Gravel Rt.
  Nervous, highly——Peppermint
  Nervous irritation—Ro. Chamomile
  Popular with Indian women—Blue Cohosh
  Spasmodic pain—Pleurisy Rt.
  Suppressed by cold or chill—Ro. Chamomile, Black Cohosh, White Horehound, Juniper, Pennyroyal, G. Rue, Serpentaria, Tansy, Thistle, Thyme, Amer. Wormseed
  Tonic, ovarian—False Unicorn

Tonic, uterus—Rue, Raspberry, False and True Unicorn, Myrrh, Witch Hazel

With debility—Peruvian Bark

Useful—Ro. Chamomile, Blue Cohosh, Gentian (European), Guaiacum, Black Horehound, Motherwort, Myrrh, Parsley, Peruvian Bark, Pleurisy Rt., Tansy

ANAESTHETIC—Loss of sense of touch or feeling as to pain

Nerves steady after—Myrrh

Sustains heart after—Myrrh

ANEMIA—Deficiency of red corpuscles causing poverty of the blood. Cannot carry enough nutrition to keep the body in good repair, causing pallor, weakness and palpitation of the heart.

see Blood, Chlorosis

Pernicious—Raw spinach juice, raw grapes, and juice.

Regenerate blood—Raw carrots, spinach, lettuce, turnip leaves, and watercress juices. Also raw fennel, asparagus, celery, dandelion, and endive.

To build up red corpuscles—raw beet juice, using roots and tops, alone or with raw carrot juice. Also raw grapes and juice.

Useful—Chickweed

ANUS—End of alimentary canal through which refuse of digestion is voided

see Rectum, Hemorrhoids

Itching and eruptions—see Eczema

Fissures (split or narrow opening)—W. Oak

Fistula—Yarrow

Prolapsus Ani (falling downward of the Rectum)—Oak, Witch Hazel, Sumach, White Poplar

Weakness—White Poplar

APOPLEXY—(A stroke)—sudden loss or impairment of consciousness and voluntary motion due to cerebral hemorrhage.

see Brain

Incipiency—Lobelia

To take pressure of blood from brain—Cayenne, Black Cohosh

Relief—Black Cohosh

APPENDICITIS—Inflammation of the vermiform appendix
If caused by constipation—warm enema of Catnip

APPETITE—Relish food or drink—*see* Debility
Improves—Balmony, Golden Seal, Iceland Moss, Motherwort, Peppermint, Wahoo, Wood Sage, Yarrow
Loss of—Barberry, Blessed Thistle
Loss of in general debility—Ro. Chamomile
Promotes—Amer. and Eur. Columbo, Eur. Gentian, Horseradish, Serpentaria, White Poplar
Promotes in slow convalescence—Amer. Centaury
Promotes in lax conditions of the stomach—White Poplar, Eur. Gentian

ARTERIES—Tubes conveying blood from the heart to all part of the body
see Blood, Heart, Hemorrhage, High Blood Pressure, Pulse, Veins, Circulation
Excitement relieved—Wild Cherry
Excitement relieved in Typhoid Fever—Yarrow
Excitement relieved soothed—Yarrow
Excitement produced—Black Pepper
Articular Rheumatism—Hops
Hardening of Arteries—Plenty of Vit. C
Undue tension relieved—Pleurisy Rt.
Rupture relieved—Yarrow

ARTHRITIS—Inflammation of joints because of deposits of inorganic calcium.
see Rheumatism, Gout, Joints
Eliminate inorganic calcium—Celery
Eliminate pain—Parsley
Prevent paroxysm (severe temporary attack)—Tansy

ASCITIS—Dropsy of the belly or peritoneum
see Dropsy
Abdominal—Dandelion
With chronic gastric torpor—Balmony
With chronic Hepatic torpor—Balmony

ASTHMA—Spasms of the windpipe or bronchial tubes, causing a sensation of choking. Often considered a nervous condition.

see Convulsions, Chest, Respiratory Organs

A simple recipe for Asthmatic Cough—Take 2 good handfuls of Coltsfoot Leaves, 1 oz. Garlic and 2 qts. water. Boil down to 3 pints. Strain, add ½ C. sugar, boil 10 min. Take ½ cup as often as necessary.

Cough—Lobelia

Dry—Balm of Gilead

Excessive expectoration—Comfrey, Myrrh

Hay Asthma—Spearmint

Humoral—Myrrh

Smoke as tobacco—Coltsfoot

Spasmodic—Asafoetida, Blue Cohosh, Lobelia, Skunk Cabbage, Wild Yam

Used in China since ancient times—Ephedra

Useful—Boneset, Chickweed, Black Cohosh, Coltsfoot, Comfrey, Elecampane, Red Elm, Horehound (White), Lobelia, Mistletoe, Mullein, Myrrh, Pleurisy Rt., Skunk Cabbage, Thyme

BACK—back pain is caused by many conditions
see Kidneys, Debility, Tardy Menstruation, Miscarriage, Nerves, Lumbago

Aching—Buchu, Gravel Rt., Juniper, Parsley, Uva Ursi

Aching in incontinence of urine—White Poplar

BARRENNESS—Weakness of the generative organs
see Pregnancy, Impotent, Sexual, Uterus

Relieved by—Catnip, False and True Unicorn Rt.

Tonic—False Unicorn

BILE—A greenish liquid secreted by the liver, stored in the gall bladder and released to aid digestion and constipation.
see Gall Bladder, Biliousness, Cholera, Jaundice

Ejects from gall bladder and ducts—Balmony, Bitter Rt., Olive Oil, Wahoo, Boneset

Ejects—Butternut

Hepatic derangements corrected in cholera—Purple Loosestrife

Promotes secretion by liver—Boneset, Culvers Rt., Dandelion, Wahoo

Skin tinged—Barberry

Cleans system of morbid secretion of bile—Balmony

Flows more freely—Barberry, Blessed Thistle, Blue Flag, Wahoo

Gall solidified—Culvers Rt.

Overflow not from gall stones—Senna

Lack, causing clay colored stools—Bitter Rt.

Sluggish in atonic dyspepsia—Horse Radish

Bile salts in the blood (cholemia)—Wahoo

Obstruction cleaned—Dandelion

BILIOUS CONDITIONS—Derangements of the biliary processes, possibly caused by excessive secretion of bile or by gall stones (calculus).

see Stomach, Liver, Bowels, Gall Bladder, Bile, Cholera, Headache, Nausea, Nerves

Liver inactive—Wahoo

Sluggish stomach and torpid bowels—White Poplar

Bilious colds—Boneset

Bilious colic—Cayenne, Wild Yam

Bilious fever—*see* Fevers

Bilious headache—Ro. Chamomile

Specific in bilious colic—Black horehound, Wild yam

With fever, liver not active enough—Culvers Rt.

In Rheumatism—Boneset

Useful—Low fat diet, Barberry, Boneset, Eur. Gentian, Black horehound, Ground ivy, Purple Loosestrife, Amer. Mandrake, Yellow Parilla, Pleurisy Rt., Senna, Blessed Thistle

BITES and STINGS

Insects such as bees, hornets, etc.—Aloes, Beth Rt., Plantain

Old remedy for poisonous bites and stings of insects—Plantain

Preventative against mosquito and gnat bites—Oil of Pennyroyal

Nettle stings—Plantain

Snake bites—Plantain, Black Cohosh, Lobelia

Remove insect stinger by scraping with tip of knife. Squeeze to release poison. Make a compress at once of 2 t. household ammonia and one glass of water. This will neutralize the poisons which make the sting painful.

Dog—Bitter Root

BLADDER—Receptacle for the urine.

see Urine, Dysuria, Mucous membrane, Kidneys, Gravel, Stones, Urethra, Urinary organs

Aching—Uva Ursi

Purulent (pus) decomposition of urine in the bladder—Corn silk

Catarrh (mucous discharges from the bladder)—Buchu, Juniper, Uva ursi, White poplar, White Pond lily, Yarrow, Corn silk

Catarrh, chronic—Buchu

Inflammation (Cystitis)—Burdock, Hollyhock, Smooth Sumach, Spearmint, Uva ursi, Yarrow, Marshmallow

Useful in stone and gravel—Clivers

To prevent gravel deposits—Uva ursi

Hemorrhage—Beth Rt.

Irritated—Buchu, Burdock, Irish moss, Sumach, Clivers

Irritated (Morbid)—Buchu

Irritated Neck—Clivers

Strengthens—Purple Loosestrife

Specific in ulcerated—Uva Ursi

Obstruction—Carrot

Weakness—Pipsissewa

Soothes—Corn silk

Stricture—Poplar, Carrot, Uva Ursi

Tonic—White Poplar

Neck tender and sensitive—Hollyhock

Useful—Carrot, Clivers, Corn silk, Gravel Rt., Hollyhock, Hyssop, Juniper, Maidenhair, Plantain, Purple Loosestrife, False Unicorn, Wood Sage

BLOOD

see Circulation, Arteries, Congestion, High blood pressure, Hemorrhages, Capillaries, Heart

Bleeding—see organ involved

Purifiers—Burdock, Oregon Grape, Blue Flag, Echinacea, Jam, Sarsaparilla, Queen's Delight, Wood Sage, Yellow Parilla, Myrrh, Blessed Thistle, Black Cohosh, Sanicle, Guaiacum, Yarrow, Poke, Motherwort, Pipsissewa

Purifier in Boils and Carbuncles—Echinacea

Purifier in Gonorrhea—Pipsissewa

Purifier in Glandular troubles—Poke

Coughing up or spitting of blood (Hemoptysis)—Yarrow, Black Horehound, Iceland Moss, Comfrey, see Lungs, Amer. Mandrake

Increase white corpuscles—Myrrh

Increase red corpuscles—Raw beet juice (using roots and tops alone or with raw carrot juice, raw grapes and raw grape juice.)

Regenerate blood—*see* Anemia

Reduce dilated blood vessels in alcoholics—Cayenne

Clotted blood—*see* Congestions—Hyssop

Passive bleeding—Purple Loosestrife

Poisoning—Chickweed, Plantain

Poisoning in parturition—Echinacea

Bile salt in the blood (cholemia)—Wahoo

Septic conditions—Echinacea

Septic conditions prevented—Myrrh

Outward flow—*see* Capillaries

In Urine (Hematuria)—Sumach, Gravel Root, Comfrey

HIGH BLOOD PRESSURE (Hypertension)—Abnormal tension of the walls of the arteries
see Arteries, Blood Purifiers, Heart

All persons with high blood pressure should lower their intake of salt and avoid all emotional upsets.

Useful—Black Cohosh, Cayenne

BOILS—A suppurating inflammatory sore forming a central core caused by a microbic infection.
see Abscesses, Carbuncles
see Blood impurity—Echinacea

Gum boil—Marshmallow

Inflammatory—Comfrey

Obstinate—Red Elm

Poultice—Red Elm

Useful—Burdock, Echinacea, Hops, Linseed, Plantain, Wood Sage

BONES—*see* Joints, Fractures, Periosteal, rickets, limbs

Poultices for broken bones—Comfrey, Boneset

Fractures—Need Vitamin K

BOWELS—the part of the alimentary canal below the stomach —intestines or entrails.
see Colitis, alvine canal, Bilious, constipation, Infant's troubles, gas

Lower—Cascara Sagrada, Butternut, Boneset

Mucous membrane—Yarrow, Hyssop, Iceland Moss, Bitter root

Griping—Ginger, Cloves

Cramps or pains—Cayenne, Bayberry

Gently cleanse—Hyssop, Barberry, Hops, Polypody

Bleeding—Mullein, Chickweed

Hemorrhage—Cranesbill, Bayberry, Beth Rt.

Tonic—Golden Seal

Flatulence—Eur Columbo

Chronic and acute inflammation or soreness—Red Elm, Chickweed, Comfrey

Nourishment—Olive Oil

Lubricates—Olive Oil

Hard and massive movements— *see* Constipation

Impaction—Olive Oil enema

Canker—Bayberry

Invagination (drawing in a portion of the wall)—Catnip

In Typhoid Fever—Asafoetida

Relaxed state (Diarrhea and Dysentery)—Red Raspberry, Sumach, Rhubarb

Strengthens—Mullein

Irritated—Marshmallow, Licorice

Nerves—Asafoetida

Muscle membranes—Bitter Rt.

Spasms—Peppermint, Asafoetida

Tuberculosis—Irish Moss

Torpid in sluggish stomach—White Poplar

Useful—Columbo, Blue Flag, Bistort, Cascara Sagrada, Wahoo, Bitter Rt., Boneset, Clivers, Butternut

BRAIN (Cerebral)—The nerve center of the body.
  see Phrenitis, Apoplexy, Nerves

Congestion—Asafoetida

Inflammation (Encephalitis)—Asafoetida

Tonic—Skullcap

Headaches in back of head and base of brain—Black Cohosh

Removes pressure of blood from brain—Cayenne, Black Cohosh

Quiets nervous excitement—Sage

Lessens cerebral excitement—Mistletoe

163

Cerebro-spinal—Boneset, *see* Meninges
Relieves brain irritation in typhoid—Lady's Slipper

BREAST—The front of the thorax in either sex; the chest; the
bosom.
see Milk

MAMMA, MAMMARY—Breast organ which secretes milk

MAMMILLA—Nipple

MASTITIS (Inflammation of female breast)—Marshmallow, Sage
Breast abscess—*see* blood purifiers
Sore nipples—Clivers

BREATH
see Respiratory organs, lungs, bronchitis, stomach, teeth,
gums
Specific for bad, offensive, or foul breath (Halitosis)—
Cloves, Myrrh, Charcoal
Breathing with difficulty—*see* Asthma
Breathing with difficulty in Pleurisy—Pleurisy Rt.
Onion or garlic smell—Parsley

BRIGHT'S DISEASE (Nephritis)—Inflammation of the kidneys.
The presence of albumin in the urine is one of the first symp-
toms of the existence of Bright's disease.
see Albuminaria, Kidneys, Urine
Useful—False Unicorn, Burdock, Marshmallow, Red Elm,
Lobelia, Pipsissiwa, Linseed
Congestions—Cubebs
Inflammation in chronic congestions—Cubebs
Tonic—*see* Kidneys
Chronic—Uva Ursi, Carrots

BRONCHITIS—Inflammation of the bronchi—either of the 2
main branches of the trachea or its ramifications.
see Coughs, Mucous Membranes, Lungs, Respiratory Or-
gans, Hemorrhage, Chest, Catarrh
With biliousness and constipation—Boneset
Coughs, spasmodic—Lobelia, Red Clover
Chronic—Iceland Moss, Irish Moss, Yellow Parilla
Acute—Pleurisy Rt.

Irritated, inflamed bronchi—Thyme, Chickweed, Maidenhair, Sanicle, Comfrey

Excessive expectoration in chronic bronchitis—Ground Ivy

Assists expectoration—Polypody

Useful—Hyssop, Pleurisy Rt., Elecampane, Maidenhair, Asafoetida, Ginger, Linseed, Lobelia, False Unicorn, Black Horehound, Skunk Cabbage, Red Elm, Coltsfoot, Wild Cherry, Mullein, Beth Rt.

BRUISES—Injury without laceration (contusions)
>
> *see* Sprains, Sores
> Useful—Mullein, Hops
> Poultice—Sassafras, White Oak, Comfrey, Roman Chamomile, Figwort
> Liniment—Cayenne
> Removes discolorations—Hyssop
> Eyes—Hyssop, Purple Loosestrife
> Wash—White Poplar

BUBOES—Inflammatory swelling of a lymphatic gland: esp. when in the groin.
> Poultice—Bayberry, Hemlock Spruce
> Irritable—Golden Seal

BURNS and SCALDS—A wound or hurt caused by burning.
> Gun Powder—Linseed
> External applications—Keep wet with raw Linseed Oil
> Useful——Olive Oil, Marshmallow, Red Elm, White Poplar, Aloes

CALCULUS—A morbid concretion (stones) formed in the gall bladder, kidneys, and other parts of the body—lime—calcareous deposits.
> *see* Stones

CANKER—Ulcerous sore, especially in the mouth.
> *see* Ulcers
> Throat—Red Raspberry
> Tongue—Red Raspberry
> Mouth—Red Raspberry
> Stomach—Bayberry, Rue
> Bowels—Bayberry

Alimentary canal (most effective)—Bistort
Mucous membrane—Red Raspberry

CAPILLARIES—Minute blood vessels
  see Circulation, Blood
  Inducing free capillary circulation—Myrrh, Vervain, Bayberry, Cayenne, Prickly Ash, Jam Sarsaparilla, Amer. Centaury, Pleurisy Rt., Guaiacum, Roman Chamomile, Hyssop, Serpentaria, Elecampane, Motherwort, Bl. Pepper, Tansy, White Horehound, Wild Yam, Red Clover, Ground Ivy, Blue Flag, Lobelia
  Sustains Circulation—Pennyroyal

CARBUNCLES—Like a boil with a tendency to spread
  see Boils, Abscesses
  Poultice—Carrot, Red Elm, Bayberry
  see blood impurities—Echinacea
  Useful—Peruvian Bark

CATARRH—Inflammation of a mucous membrane accompanied by an abnormal discharge of mucous.
  see Coughs, Fevers, Colds, Gastric, Expectoration, Grippe, Phthisis, *see* organ involved
  Bloody mucus—Iceland Moss
  Gastric membrane—Golden Seal
  Pulmonic—Pleurisy Rt.
  Acute—Pleurisy Rt.
  Bronchial—Pleurisy Rt., Elecampane, Blue Cohosh, Asafoetida
  Chronic in aged—Hyssop
  Chronic—Elecampane, Iceland Moss, Myrrh, Hyssop, Skunk Cabbage
  Respiratory organs—Polypody Rt., Bl. Horehound, White Horehound
  Cystic—Cubebs, Corn Silk, Pipsissewa, Buchu, Juniper, White Poplar, Uva Ursi, Maiden Hair, Plantain, White Pond Lily
  Chronic Cystic inflammation—Cubebs
  Intestinal—Horseradish
  Dyspepsia—Elecampane
  Wet—White Horehound, Wild Cherry
  Infants—Asafoetida
  Cough—Mullein, Blue Cohosh

When expectoration is difficult of removal—Polypody
Epidemic (influenza)—Boneset
Ophthalmia—Cranesbill
Useful—Pleurisy Rt., Boneset, Spearmint, White Horehound,
    Licorice, Wild Cherry, Mullein, Maidenhair, Asafoetida,
    Sanicle, Linseed, Amer. Mandrake

CERVIX—Any neck-like part; the neck
    see Uterus, Neck
    Ulcerated—White Pond Lily

CHANCRE—The initial lesion of syphilis, commonly a more or
    less distinct ulcer or sore with a hard base
    see Syphilis, Venereal
    Irritable—Golden Seal
    Excoriation and chancre of prepuce and vulva—White Pond
    Lily

CHARCOAL
    Anti-acid for stomach acidity—removes heartburn
    Useful on ulcers, to remove offensive odors from intestinal or
    kidney discharges, water brash, and from the feet.
    Useful to check decay, purify the breath, in nausea and
    vomiting, and in fermentative dyspepsia
    Valuable in the incipient stages of consumption.

CHEST DISEASES—(The Thorax)—Trunk of the body from the
    neck to belly.
    see Asthma, Bronchitis, Pleurisy, Pneumonia, Colds, Heart,
    Fevers, Lungs
    Irritated—Hollyhock
    Excessive and difficult expectoration—Polypody, Myrrh
    Sore—Mullein
    Useful—Pleurisy Rt., Asafoetida, Hyssop, Licorice, Wild
    Cherry, Mullein, Chickweed, Elecampane

CHILBLAINS—A blain, sore or inflammation produced on the
    hands or feet by exposure to cold.
    If not open, exterior—Red Elm
    Washing with the water in which potatoes were boiled
    (certainly he means without salt) as hot as can be borne.
    This should give immediate relief.

CHILLS—Coldness, usually with shivering
  see Ague, Colds
  Arrest—Peppermint, Senna
  Useful—Ginger, Cayenne, Lobelia·
  Congestive—Bl. Pepper

CHLOROSIS—"Green Sickness"—A form of anemia
  see Anemia, blood purifiers
  see Blood impurity—Motherwort
  Hysteria—Motherwort
  Heart palpitation—Motherwort
  Scrofulous impurity—Motherwort
  Useful—Myrrh

CHOLERA—Bilious disease—generally marked by profuse purg-
    ing, vomiting, cramps
  see Bile, bilious conditions
  Useful—Cayenne, Purple Loosestrife, Bistort, Peppermint
  Stomach irritated—Purple Loosestrife
  Hepatic dearrangement—Purple Loosestrife

CHOLERA INFANTUM (Cholera in Infants)—see Cholera
  Useful—Peppermint, Cayenne, Linseed, Purple Loosestrife,
    White Poplar, Eur. Columbo, Oak, Rhubarb, Red Elm
  Severe cases—Cranesbill
  Secondary stage—Rhubarb

CHOLERA MORBUS (Sporadic Cholera in Infants)—see Cholera
  Useful—Purple Loosestrife, Eur. Columbo, Wild Yam

CHOREA—A nervous disease marked by irregular and involun-
    tary convulsions of the muscles, esp. of the face and limbs
    —(St. Vitus Dance).
  see Nerves, Convulsions
  Specific—Skullcap, Black Cohosh
  Useful—Blue and Black Cohosh, Skunk Cabbage, Mistletoe,
    Peruvian Bark
  With debility—Peruvian Bark

CIRCULATION—Movement of the blood through the various
    vessels of the body
  see Arteries, Blood, Capillaries, Portal

Failing—Cayenne

Sluggish—Blue Flag, Prickly Ash, Ginger, Cayenne, Bayberry

Equalizes—Cayenne, Lobelia, Yarrow, Bayberry, Myrrh, Black Cohosh

Stimulates—Yellow Parilla, Cubebs, Eur. Gentian, Myrrh, Horseradish, Balm of Gilead, Cayenne, Catnip, Blessed Thistle, Bayberry, Black Pepper, Guaiacum, Rue

Arterial—Prickly Ash, Serpentaria, Bayberry, Cayenne

Cleans of Urea—Corn Silk

Tonic—Myrrh

In parturition, it equalizes the circulation—Serpentaria

Scrofula—*see* blood purifiers

Interrupted—*see* Gangrene

Venous tonic—Golden Seal, Eur. Gentian

COLDS

see Lungs, Respiratory, Chest, Chills, Coughs, Dysmenorrhea, Ammenorrhea, Pulmonary troubles, fever, catarrh, hoarseness

In nasal passages—*see* Nose

In infants—W. Horehound

In head—Sanicle, Vinegar

In stomach—Cayenne, Carrot

Exceedingly valuable—White Horehound

Useful—Pennyroyal, Yarrow, Peppermint, Lobelia, Comfrey, Tansy, Red Elm, Pleurisy Rt., Boneset, Bayberry, Vervain, Cayenne, Linseed, White Horehound, Ginger, Hyssop, Wood Sage, Thyme, Roman Chamomile, Catnip, Blessed Thistle, Marshmallow, Coltsfoot, Asafoetida, Pipsissiwa, Hemlock Spruce, Maidenhair, Black Pepper

Feet cold during parturition—Serpentaria

Congestive chill—Black Pepper

Irritable cold—Hollyhock

Extremities are cold—Prickly Ash

With biliousness and constipation—Boneset

COLIC—Spasmodic cramping or convulsion of the intestines, esp. of the large intestine, causing violent pain, caused usually by fermentation of food in the intestine.

see Gas, Spasms, Stomach

Bilious—Cayenne, Wild Yam

Specific in bilious colic—Bl. Horehound, Wild Yam—check Liver and Bile

Griping—Ginger, Cloves

Children—Catnip

Useful—Thyme, Spearmint, Valerian, Lady's Slipper, Pennyroyal, Peppermint, Wild Yam, Blue Cohosh, Bayberry, G. Rue, Ginger

Painter's or Lead Poisoning—Ground Ivy, Red Elm

Flatulent—Ginger, Asafoetida

COLITIS—Inflammation of the mucous membrane of the colon— *see* Bowels, Alvine Canal

Nutritious—Olive Oil, Red Elm

COMA—A state of prolonged unconsciousness.

From narcotic poisoning—Coffee, Bayberry, Lobelia emetic

Useful—Lobelia

CONGESTION (Hyperaemia)—An unnatural accumulation of blood in the vessels of an organ or part

see Organ involved, Chills, Colds, Cystic, Dysmenorrhea, Amenorrhea.

Useful—Ginger, White Horehound, Sassafras, Bayberry, Cayenne

With nervous irritation—Lady's Slipper

Of the lungs—White Horehound

Of the Uterus—Wild Yam

CONJUNCTIVA—CONJUNCTIVITIS—The mucous membrane which lines the inner surface of the eyelids.

see Eyes, Trachoma

A good wash—Witch Hazel

Granular—Poke

CONSTIPATION—Incomplete or inadequate action of the bowels.

see Bowels, Headache, Nerves, Bile

Lower Bowel at fault—Cascara Sagrada, Butternut, Boneset

Assisting peristaltic action—Cayenne, Cascara Sagrada, Butternut, Senna

Causing Appendicitis—warm enema of Catnip

Chronic—Cascara Sagrada, Culver's Rt., Senna, Butternut, Blue Flag, Balmony, Oregon Grape

Habitual—Olive Oil, Wahoo, Cascara Sagrada, Butternut,
Habitual with torpor of digestive organs—Aloes
With flatulence—Asafoetida
In colds, bronchitis and pneumonia—Boneset
In dyspeptic—Boneset, Rhubarb
In inactivity of liver—Wahoo
Impaction—Olive Oil
Liver and bowels need help—Boneset
With torpid stomach and liver—Horseradish, Wahoo
Badly constipated—Yarrow
With uterine atony—Aloes
Hard, dry, massive feces—Olive Oil, Golden Seal
Useful—Aloes, Poke, Blessed Thistle, Dandelion, Red Elm,
   Barberry, Cayenne, Balmony, Boneset, Queens Delight,
   Blue Flag, Purple Loosestrife, Red Raspberry, Senna,
   Ginger
Mild laxatives—Barberry, Olive Oil, Hops, Red Clover, Poly-
   pody, Cascara Sagrada

CONVALESCENCE—After illness, to make progress toward re-
   covery of health
   see Fevers, Nerves, Debility, Tonics
   Nourishing—Red Raspberry
   Promotes appetite—Amer. Centaury
   From debilitating diseases—Vervain, Eur. Columbo
   From idiopathic fevers—Roman Chamomile
   Hastens after pregnancy—Red Raspberry
   From typhoid—Amer. Columbo
   Slow—Amer. Centaury

CONVULSIONS—Violent and involuntary spasmodic contraction
   of the muscles
   see Spasms, Asthma, Epilepsy, Respiratory, Nerves, Hys-
   teria, Coughs, Cramps, Fits, St. Vitus Dance
   In children—Catnip, G. Rue
   Puerperal—Assist flow during convulsions—Blue Cohosh,
   Skullcap, Black Cohosh, Lobelia
   Infantile—Asafoetida, Peppermint, Valerian, Lobelia, Catnip,
   Rue
   Adults—G. Rue, Mistletoe, Cramp Bark, Vervain, Skullcap,
   Peppermint, Lobelia, Asafoetida, Valerian, Blue Cohosh

COUGHS—*see* Asthma, Bronchitis, Catarrh, Lungs, Whooping
Coughs, Expectoration, Respiratory Organs
Useful—Wild Cherry, Black Cohosh, Licorice, White and
Black Horehound, Red Elm, Comfrey, Elecampane, Pip-
sissiwa, Ground Ivy, Hyssop, Lobelia, Vervain, Marshmal-
low, Iceland Moss, Coltsfoot, Mullein, Maidenhair, Blue
Cohosh, Linseed, Amer. Mandrake, Roman Chamomile,
Beth Rt., Polypody.
Children's and infant's—Lobelia, Asafoetida, W. Horehound
Colds—Mullein, Maidenhair
Colds, bilious—Boneset
Dry, irritable, hacking—Hollyhock
Croupy—Mullein
In the aged—White Horehound
Old—Balm of Gilead
Irritable tickling—Hyssop
Irritable—Hops, Maidenhair, Wild Cherry, Skunk Cabbage
Persistent tickling—Licorice
Chronic—Irish Moss, Pleurisy Rt., Coltsfoot, Boneset
Diminish mucous discharges—Myrrh
Nervous—Wild Cherry, Lobelia, Asafoetida, Comfrey
Hysteria—Lobelia
Acute—Wild Cherry
Infant suffocating from phlegm—Lobelia
With torpid liver—Wahoo
Convulsive coughs in Tuberculosis—Black Cohosh

WHOOPING COUGH (Pertussis)—A paroxysmal cough, gen-
erally infectious. *see* Cough, Expectoration
Specific—Thyme
Useful—Black and Blue Cohosh, Skunk Cabbage, Elecam-
pane, Coltsfoot, Wild Cherry, Asafoetida, Lobelia, Red
Clover

CRAMPS—*see* Convulsions, Spasms
Bowels—Cayenne, Bayberry
All kinds—Cramp Bark, Cayenne, Valerian, Lobelia, Blue
Cohosh, Wild Yam
In pregnancy—Cramp Bark, Wild Yam
Spasmodic in cholera—Purple Loosestrife
Stomach—Bayberry

CROUP—*see* Diphtheria
   In children and infants—White Horehound, Lobelia
   Useful—Asafoetida, Lobelia
   Throat sore and inflamed after false membrane has been
      cleared out—Red Elm, Pineapple
   Cough—Mullein
   Membraneous Croup—Pleurisy Rt., Lobelia
   Mucus Croup—Lobelia
   Spasmodic—Lobelia

CUTANEOUS—affecting skin
   see Eczema, Skin, Psoriasis, Shingles, Tetters, Eruptions
   Cutaneous eruptions—Figwort, Guaiacum, Buchu, Poke, Yel-
      low Parilla, Juniper, Pipsissewa
   Eruptions with strumous diathesis—Pipsissewa
   Obstinate cutaneous eruptions—Olive Oil, Peruvian Bark,
      Queen's Delight

CYSTIC—Closed bladder-like sac containing fluid or semi-fluid
      morbid matter.
   see Catarrh
   Inflammation—Corn silk
   Congestion—Cubebs, White Poplar

DEAFNESS—Impervious to sound.
   see Ear
   Caused by too much quinine or Peruvian Bark

DEBILITY (Asthenic)—Weak or feeble
   see Tonics, Convalescence, Exhaustion, Dropsy, Fainting,
      Prostration, Digestion, Appetite, Nerves, Back, Stomach
   In alimentary canal—Eur., Columbo, Ginger
   Of the digestive organs—Elecampane, *Iceland Moss, Eu-
      ropean Gentian, Horseradish*
   Of female generative system—Poplar, True Unicorn
   Female and male weakness—Skullcap
   In acute disease—Iceland Moss
   Pelvic weakness—Gravel Root, Thistle
   Chronic catarrh in aged—Hyssop
   General debility—Balmony, White Poplar, Peruvian Bark,
      Tansy, Amer. and Eur. Gentian, Yellow Parilla, Hops,
      Roman Chamomile, Catnip, White Horehound, Iceland

Moss, Pomgranate. Hyssop, Red Elm, Irish Moss, Guaiacum, Oak, Asafoet .a, Amer. Centaury, Lobelia, Vervain,
Columbo, Chickweed, Wild Cherry, Cayenne, Dandelion,
Horseradish, Pipsissewa, Myrrh, Boneset, Blue Flag, Elecampane

Lungs (Pulmonary)—Balm of Gilead
Lymphatic—Blue Flag
Kidneys—Tansy
Scrofulous—Pipsissewa, Blue Flag, Peruvian Bark
Mucous membrane—Golden Seal, Hyssop, Guaiacum
In large purulent discharges—Iceland Moss, Peruvian Bark
In old age—White Poplar, Hyssop, Red Elm, Bayberry
Sinking spells—Cayenne
For energy—Take dessiccated Liver
Overworked and worried—Lady's Slipper
Chronic diseases—Peruvian Bark
Hemorrhages—Peruvian Bark
Fed through rectum—Olive Oil
Nervous Prostration—Lady's Slipper, Skullcap, Yarrow
Spasms from weakness—Peruvian Bark

DELIRIUM—Temporary disorder of the mental faculties
    see Nerves, Fevers
In Typhoid—Lady's Slipper, Skullcap
Alcoholic—Hops
Delirium Tremens—a wine-glassful of strong vinegar will
    soon restore sense and locomotion: Skullcap, Hops, Lo-
    belia
Nerves quieted—Hops, Motherwort, Vervain, Sage, Skull-
    cap, Lady's Slipper, Mistletoe

DIABETES

DIABETES INSIPIDUS—Persistent abnormally large discharge
    of urine

DIABETES MELLITUS—Excessive amount of sugar in the urine
    Useful—Hollyhock, Smooth Sumach, False Unicorn

DIARRHEA—Frequent discharge of loose fecal matter from
    the bowels
    see Dysentery
Acute—White Oak, White Poplar, Beth Rt.

Useful—Butternut, Cranesbill, Red Raspberry, Culvers Rt., Eur. Gentian, Comfrey, Plantain, Tormentil, Purple Loosestrife, Marshmallow, Hemlock Spruce, Oak, Eur. Columbo, Witch Hazel, Ginger, Amer. Columbo, Mullein, Sanicle, Bayberry, Bistort, White Pond Lily, Linseed, Pomegranate

Highly recommended—Red Elm, Rhubarb

Scrofulous—Plantain, Pipsissewa

In typhoid—Amer. Columbo

Infants and children—Black Cohosh, Rhubarb

Bleeding bowels—Mullein

Chronic—Sumach, Catechu, White Poplar, Yarrow, Oak, Iceland Moss, Beth Rt.

Caused by intestinal irritation—Red Elm

DIGESTIVE ORGANS—*see* Tonics, Digestion, Indigestion, Intestinal

Debilitated—Iceland Moss, Eur. Gentian, Elecampane

Weakness—Eur. Gentian, Golden Seal, Elecampane, Mistletoe

Torpid conditions—Wahoo

Torpid with constipation—Aloes

Invigorating digestive function—Amer. Centaury

Tonic—Uva Ursi, Barberry, Eur. Gentian, Yarrow

Atonic and depressed conditions—Wild Cherry

Useful—Cubebs, Guaiacum

Enfeebled in dropsy—Horseradish

Derangement—Dandelion

DIGESTION—*see* Digestive Organs, Tonic, Indigestion, Bile, Dyspepsia

Weak—Eur. Gentian, Amer. and Eur. Columbo, Roman Chamomile

Assists—Golden Seal, Motherwort, Rhubarb, Wahoo, Horseradish, Cloves, Bl. Pepper, Serpentaria, Eur. Gentian, Roman Chamomile, Iceland Moss, Tansy, Cayenne

Weakness from lax condition of stomach—White Poplar, Eur. Gentian

Digestion upset when bile is absorbed and skin tinged—Barberry

Atonic and depressed conditions—Wild Cherry

Improves gastric and intestinal digestion—Motherwort

Disordered digestion—Pipsissewa
Weak in infants—Rhubarb, Cod Liver Oil
Regurgitation of food—Bl. Horehound

DIPHTHERIA—*see* Croup, Mucous Membrane
Sore Throat—Sumach, Myrrh, Cayenne, Oak, Red Elm, Pineapple, Lemon
Neck compress of tincture of Cayenne
With putrescence—Cayenne
Useful—Myrrh, Cayenne

DIZZINESS
Useful—Peppermint

DROPSY—An excessive accumulation of serous fluid
see Urine, Ascitis, Kidneys
In chronic engorgement of abdominal viscera—Elecampane
Kidney tonic—Parsley, Pipsissewa
Useful—Blessed Thistle, Amer. Mandrake, Juniper, Bl. Horehound, Horseradish, Skunk Cabbage, Mullein, Black Cohosh, Wahoo, Burdock, Blue Flag, Dandelion, Peruvian Bark, Gravel Rt., Clivers, Buchu, Parsley, Carrot, Bitter Rt., Pipsissewa
see Blood Purifier
Cardiac (Heart)—Bitter Rt.
With chronic hepatic and gastric torpor—Balmony
Debilitated system—Horseradish, Peruvian Bark
Cellular—Mullein
Synovial—Mullein
Digestive organs enfeebled—Horseradish
Abdominal—Dandelion
Dropsied limbs—Mullein

DYSENTERY—An infectious disease characterized by inflammation and ulceration of the lower portion of the bowels, with diarrhea that soon becomes mucous and hemorrhagic.
see Diarrhea, Bowels
Useful—Sumach, Culvers Rt., Cranesbill, Bayberry, Witch Hazel, Rhubarb, Cayenne, Butternut, Oak, Linseed, Sanicle, Beth Rt., Yarrow, Mullein, White and Yellow Pond Lily, Eur. Columbo, Pleurisy Rt., Comfrey, Marshmallow, Red Elm, Purple Loosestrife, Red Raspberry, Bistort, Ginger

176

Chronic—Yarrow, Rhubarb, White Poplar, Iceland Moss, Cranesbill, Pomegranate, Purple Loosestrife

Scrofulous—Plantain, Pipsissewa

DYSMENORRHEA—Difficult or painful menstruation
see Menstruation, Cold

Useful—Black and Blue Cohosh, Poke, Wild Yam, Hemlock Spruce, True Unicorn, Valerian, Bl. Horehound, Pleurisy Rt., Lady's Slipper, Asafoetida, Parsley, Roman Chamomile, Motherwort, Hops

Causing irritated nerves—Roman Chamomile, Pennyroyal

Antispasmodic—Pleurisy Rt.

With congestion—Motherwort

DYSPEPSIA (Indigestion)—*see* Indigestion, Digestion

Useful—American Centaury, Balmony, Dandelion, Blessed Thistle, Golden Seal, Cayenne, Wild Cherry, Yarrow, Poke, Hops, Lobelia, Ginger, Peruvian Bark, Eur. Columbo, Serpentaria, Iceland Moss, Amer. and Eur. Gentian, Boneset, Peruvian Bark

Chronic—Cascara Bark, Amer. Mandrake

Atonic—Yellow Parilla

Atonic with sluggish bile—Horseradish

Tonic—False Unicorn, Wahoo

Fermentative dyspepsia—Echinacea, Charcoal

Congested liver—Dandelion, Senna, Butternut

Congested Spleen—Culvers Root, American Mandrake

During pregnancy—True Unicorn

Nervous—Skullcap

Catarrhal—Elecampane

With foul breath and gaseous eructation—Cloves, Myrrh

Gas with pain—Cayenne

With constipation—Boneset, Rhubarb

Torpor with constipation—Aloes

DYSURIA—Difficult or painful urination
see Urine, Stranguria, Bladder, Micturition, Kidneys

Tonic—White Poplar

EARS—*see* Deafness

Noises—Too much Quinine or Peruvian Bark

Inflammation (OTITIS)—Lobelia

ECZEMA—An inflammatory disease of the skin attended with itching and the exudation of serous matter.
 see Cutaneous, Eruptions, Skin, Tetters
 Useful—Burdock, Golden Seal, Olive Oil, Plantain, Oregon Grape, Queen's Delight, Guaiacum, Onion poultice
 Wash—White Poplar
 Specific—Burdock

EMPHYSEMA—Air in the interstices of the connective tissue, usually through atrophy of the septa between the alveoli.
 see Lungs
 Useful—Cheken

EPILEPSY—A nervous disease characterized by recurrent attacks of more or less severe convulsions, usually attended by loss of consciousness.
 see Spasms
 Useful—Black Cohosh, Lobelia, Skullcap, Mistletoe, Valerian
 Convulsions at regular intervals—Peruvian Bark

ERUPTIONS or ERUPTIVE DISEASES—Outbreak like a rash
 see Eczemas, Skin, Cutaneous, Face, Smallpox, Impetigo, Measles, Pimples, Erysipelas, Psoriasis, Shingles, Scarlet Fever
 Acne—*see* Blood Purifiers
 Irritation—*see* Skin
 Nettle Rash—Sanicle, Serpentaria, Plantain
 Tardy eruptions or receded—Serpentaria
 Hastens in measles—Yarrow
 Hastens eruptions—Pennyroyal, Yarrow, Serpentaria
 Useful—Pleurisy Rt., Ginger, Chickweed, Ground Ivy, Hyssop, Black Cohosh, Culvers Rt., Senna, Burdock, Jam Sarsaparilla, Sassafras, Queen's Delight, Serpentaria, Sanicle
 Fever in eruptive diseases—Sanicle, Ginger
 see Blood Purifiers
 From heptic torpor—Wahoo
 Contagious—Sassafras
 Itching—Golden Seal
 Burning sensation—Golden Seal
 Scabs on hands and heads of children—Spearmint
 Prevent scales from spreading from patient—Golden Seal

ERYSIPELAS (St. Anthony's Fire)—An acute, febrile, infectious
disease, due to a specific streptococcus and characterized
by a diffusely spreading, deep red inflammation of the
skin or mucous membrane.
  see Eruptions, Skin
  Useful—Plantain, Golden Seal, Echinacea
  Severe cases relieved—Chickweed
  Gangrenous—Peruvian Bark

EXHAUSTION (Prostration)—Extreme weakness or fatigue
  see Debility, Fainting, Heat, Sunstroke, Nerves
  Specific for overheat—Pennyroyal
  Useful—Bl. Pepper
  Nervous—Celery, Skullcap, Yarrow
  Nervous, profound—Skullcap

EXPECTORATION—Expels phlegm or mucus
  see Catarrh, Coughs, Respiratory Organs, Chest, Whoop-
  ing Cough, Phlegm, Phthisis
  Useful—Coltsfoot
  Debilitating—Iceland Moss
  Excessive—Iceland Moss, Comfrey, Hyssop
  Excessive in Tuberculosis—Myrrh, Yellow Parilla
  Difficult of removal—Polypody, Myrrh
  Purulent expectoration—Iceland Moss
  Bronchi—Polypody
  Bloody (Hemoptysis)—Iceland Moss
  Bloody in asthma—Comfrey, Myrrh
  In lung troubles—W. Horehound, Elecampane, Pleurisy Rt.

EYES—*see* Conjunctiva, Ophthalmia
  Inflammation—Golden Seal, Marshmallow, Witch Hazel
  Ulceration of the cornea—Golden Seal
  Clouded vision, if crystalline humour is not injured or
  destroyed—Purple Loosestrife
  Preserving the sight—Purple Loosestrife
  Double vision—Asafoetida
  Ulceration of the cornea in granular opthalmia—Golden Seal
  Yellow vision—*see* Jaundice
  Black (bruised) eye—Hyssop, Purple Loosestrife
  Sore—White Pond Lily, Golden Seal, Parsley
  Protrusion of the eyeball—*see* Goitre (Exophthalmic)

Hayfever—Mullein
Violent pains—Peruvian Bark

FACE—*see* Eruptions, Mumps
Neuralgia—Skullcap, Wild Yam
Acne—*see* Blood Purifiers
Removes wrinkles—Myrrh
Violent pains—Peruvian Bark
Freckles—wash with cucumbers

FAINTING—Extreme weakness or exhaustion
see Tonics, Debility, Exhaustion
Useful—Cramp Bark, White Poplar, Lobelia

FAUCES—Cavity at the back of the mouth, leading into the
pharynx
see Thrush, Mouth, Pharyngitis
Useful—Lobelia
Paralysis—Ginger
Inflammation—White Oak

FEET—*see* Chilblains, Felon, Whitlow, Gout, Skin, Limbs
Bunions—Poke
Cold from sluggish circulation—Cayenne, Prickly Ash
Cold during partuition—Serpentaria
Sweaty and tender—White Oak
Foot bath in tardy menses—Mustard, Cayenne, Ginger
Offensive odors—Charcoal

FELON—Acute and painful inflammation of the deeper tissues
of a finger or toe, usually near the nail.
see Feet, Whitlow
Poultices—Poke
Slip your finger into a hole cut in a lemon

FEVERS—A morbid condition of the body characterized by un-
due rise of temperature
see Convalescence, Catarrh, Chest, Delirium, Rheumatic,
Hepatic, Scarlet, Typhoid, Typhus, Yellow, Nerves, In-
flammation, Malaria, Smallpox
All forms of Fevers—Barberry, Mistletoe, Serpentaria, Sage,
Lobelia, Pleurisy Rt., Pipsissewa, Peppermint, Boneset,
Ginger, Vervain, Catnip, Hyssop, Peruvian Bark, Penny-

royal, Cayenne, Yarrow, Echinacea, Gravel Rt., Clivers,
Wood Sage, Roman Chamomile, Senna, Purple Loosestrife,
Bayberry, Amer. Centaury, Tansy, Thyme, Black Pepper

Lung fever—Pleurisy Rt.

With depressed or low vitality—Catnip

From colds—Sanicle, Catnip

Cold in respiratory tract—Sanicle

Cold in head—Sanicle

Fevers in measles—Sanicle

Fevers in Eruptive diseases—Sanicle, Ginger

Remittent (see Ague and Malaria)—Boneset, Blessed Thistle, Senna, Eur. Columbo, Roman Chamomile, Amer. Centaury, Pleurisy Rt., Culvers Rt.

Intermittent (see Ague and Malaria)—Boneset, Tansy, Blessed Thistle, Senna, Wild Cherry, Valerian, Roman Chamomile, Peruvian Bark, Black Pepper, Oak, Pomegranate,
Amer. Centaury, Bl. Pepper, Serpentaria, Eur. Gentian

Convalescence from idiopathic disease—Roman Chamomile

Acute fevers—Culvers Rt., Bayberry

Bilious—Ro. Chamomile, Pleurisy Rt., Boneset

Low with restlessness—Valerian

Spotted—see Meninges

Low, with or without inflammation, suppurative or gangrenous—Peruvian Bark

Lingering—Hyssop

Yellow fever—Cayenne, Boneset, see Jaundice

Breakbone (influenza)—Boneset, see Grippe

Prevent—Boneset

Bilious remitting—Boneset

Black or slow fever—Lobelia

Thirst quenched—Sumach, Strawberry, Lemon, White, Red
and Black Mulberry, Red Currant, Pomegranate

Tonic in convalescence—Yarrow, Wild Cherry, Eur. Columbo,
Motherwort, Skullcap, Vervain

Puerperal—Lobelia, Pleurisy Rt., Roman Chamomile

Nervous excitement—Motherwort

Delirium—Lady's Slipper, Sage, Skullcap, Bl. Pepper, Vervain, Hops, Mistletoe

Hectic fever—Sage, Pomegranate

Hectic fever in consumption—Wild Cherry

Hectic fever in phthisis—Eur. Columbo
Hectic fever in scrofula—Wild Cherry
Hectic fever with exhaustive sweats—Sage, Pomegranate
Urine scanty, with or without brick dust deposits—Gravel Rt.
Liver not active enough in Thyphoid, Typhus, Bilious, Re-
mitting, Rheumatic Fevers, and others—Culvers Rt.
Restlessness—*see* Sleep
Nervous and cross children—*see* Infants
In place of Peruvian Bark or Quinine—W. Poplar

FITS—A sudden morbid seizure characterized by loss of consciousness or by convulsions.
see Convulsions, Epilepsy

FLATULENT—Suffering from an accumulation of gas
see Gas, Alimentary Canal
Useful—Bl. Pepper, Ginger, Carrots, Charcoal, Pleurisy Rt.,
Peppermint, Rue, Thyme, Cloves, Pennyroyal, Wild Yam,
Cayenne, Spearmint
Prevent—Peppermint
Griping—Ginger, Cloves
Relieve in atonic indigestion—Myrrh
In the bowels with constipation—Asafoetida
In the bowels—Eur. Columbo
In debilitated stomach—Sage
With pain in dyspepsia—Charcoal, Cayenne
Fermentative dyspepsia—Echinacea
Stomach—Cramp Bark, Pleurisy Rt, Cayenne
With uterine atony—Aloes

GALL BLADDER and DUCTS—*see* Bile, Bilious conditions,
Liver, Hepatics, Stones
Stimulates Gall Ducts, influencing excretion of bile—Bitter
Rt., Wahoo, Boneset
Relieves engorgement of gall ducts—Senna
Relieves gall ducts—Horseradish, Blue Flag
Relaxing to gall ducts—Hops
Liquifies gall (bile) in relief of gall stones—Amer. Mandrake
Useful in gall stones—Olive Oil, Bitter Rt., Parsley, Dande-
lion, Roman Chamomile
Tonic to Gall Ducts—Rhubarb

Useful—Cascara Sagrada, Yellow Parilla, Blessed Thistle, Purple Loosestrife, Amer. Mandrake
Occlusion of the gall ducts—Lobelia
Pains and nerves of gall stones—Wild Yam
Clay-colored stools—Bitter Rt.
Influencing liver to secret bile (but not excretion through gall ducts)—Culvers Rt.—*see* Bile
Influences liver to secrete bile and to excrete from gall ducts—Wahoo. *see* Bile

GANGRENE—The dying of tissue, as from interruption of circulation.
see Circulation
Sores—Bayberry, Cayenne, Marshmallow
Useful—Echinacea, Marshmallow, Wood Sage, Oak, Peruvian Bark
Ulcers—Carrot

GAS—*see* Flatulent, Bowels, Colic
Gaseous eructation—Charcoal
Useful—Pennyroyal, G. Rue
Poisoning (World War I)—Lily of the Valley

GASTRIC—Of, or pertaining to, the stomach.
see Stomach
Catarrh—Cayenne, Horseradish, Amer. Columbo, Golden Seal
Arouses warmth—Bl. Pepper
Ulcers—Amer. Columbo, Golden Seal, Red Elm, Cranesbill
Irritation—Golden Seal, Asafoetida
Improves gastric digestion—Motherwort, Wahoo
Tonic in pregnancy—False Unicorn
Chronic torpor in dropsy—Balmony
Hemorrhage—*see* Stomach
Gastric secretion aroused—Balmony

GASTRIC MEMBRANE—*see* Ulcers
Catarrh—Golden Seal
Tonic—Wahoo, Elecampane
Tonic in dyspepsia—Wahoo
Arouses gastric secretions—Balmony
Irritation—Asafoetida
Clogged with congested mucus—Golden Seal

GASTRITIS—Inflammation of the stomach, especially of its mucous membrane.
>*see* Stomach, Mucous Membrane
>Food—Red Elm
>Soothing and healing—Red Elm
>Chronic—Wild Cherry

GENERATIVE ORGANS (reproductive organs)—Having the power of reproduction.
>*see* Uterus, Ovaries, Sex, Genital Organs, Impotent, Leucorrhea, Barrenness
>Debility of the female—White Poplar, True Unicorn
>Useful—Blue Cohosh, Columbo, True Unicorn
>Tonic to mucous membrane—Beth Root, Uva Ursi
>Tonic—Amer. Centaury, Buchu, Golden Seal, Figwort, True Unicorn, False Unicorn, Yarrow, Motherwort
>Female and male weakness—False Unicorn
>Tonic to female nerves—Wild Yam
>Sterility—False Unicorn, True Unicorn
>Organs painful in female—Blue Cohosh

GENITAL ORGANS—Organs of generation (external) usually of the male
>*see* Generative Organs
>Useful—Guaiacum
>Influences mucous membrane—Beth Root, Uva Ursi
>Blood diseases—Oregon Grape. *see* Blood Purifiers
>Burning and itching—Chickweed, Tansy

GLANDS—*see* Lymphatics, Saliva, Sebaceous, Prostate, Goitre, Mucous Membrane, Mumps, Thyroid, Secernments
>Swellings, inflammations, enlarged—Yellow Parilla, Wild Meadow Sage, Mullein, Poke
>Useful—Blue Flag, Queen's Delight, Bayberry, Plantain, Pipsissewa, Lobelia, Yarrow, Mullein, Poke, Sassafras
>*see* Blood puriifiers—Poke

GLEET—Morbid discharge from the urethra
>Useful—Cranesbill, Yarrow, False Unicorn, Cubebs, Witch Hazel, Uva Ursi, White Pond Lily, Buchu

GOITRE—Morbid enlargement of the thyroid gland
>*see* Glands, Thyroid

Useful—Oak, Blue Flag, Poke, Bayberry

GONORRHEA (Clap)—A contagious, purulent inflammation of
the urethra or the vagina due to the gonococcus
see Urethra, Vagina, Venereal
Chronic—White Poplar, Gravel Rt.
Acute—Gravel Rt., Clivers
Inflammatory stage—Clivers
Lingering in females—Uva Ursi
Useful—Uva Ursi, Cubebs, Witch Hazel, Marshmallow, Hol-
lyhock, Pipsissewa, Red Raspberry
Soothes mucous membrane—Pipsissewa
Soothes nervous system—Clivers
Cleansing to the blood current—Pipsissewa. *see* Blood Puri-
fiers
Painful erections—Hops
Wash—Golden Seal

GOUT—A disease characterized by painful inflammation of the
joints (chiefly those in the feet and hands, esp. in the great
toe) and by excess uric acid in the blood (Lithaemia).
see Joints, Arthritis, Blood Purifiers
Useful—Guaiacum, Eur. Gentian, Burdock, Jam Sarsaparilla,
Dandelion, Sassafras
Acute—Wood Sage
Atonic—Ginger, Cayenne
Rheumatism—Boneset

GRAVEL—Small calculi formed in the kidneys.
see Stones, Kidneys, Bladder, Urine
One of the best—Gravel Rt.
Useful—Clivers, Uva Ursi, Marshmallow, Buchu, Juniper,
Parsley, Bl. Horehound, Carrot, Comfrey, Dandelion
To prevent—Uva Ursi.

GRIPPE—Influenza or Breakbone fever
see Catarrh, Fever, Respiratory Organs
Useful—Peppermint, Pleurisy Rt., Yarrow
"Breakbone Fever"—Boneset
Excellent—Boneset
Old remedy—Elder and Peppermint, Bayberry

185

GROWTHS—A morbid mass of tissue as a tumor.
  see Tumors, Warts, Moles
  Inflamed—Red Elm, W. Pond Lily

GUMS—see Toothache, Teeth, Breath, Scurvy
  Strengthens—Pomegranate
  Relieve toothache—rub Cloves on gums
  Spongy and inflamed—Myrrh, Hemlock Spruce, Red Raspberry, Bayberry, Oak, Smooth Sumach, Cranesbill
  Boil—Marshmallow
  Ulcerated—Bistort
  Hardens gums prior to fitting for false teeth—Oak
  Sore—Cranesbill, White Pond Lily, Witch Hazel, Bistort
  Bleeding—Oak, Bayberry

HAIR—see Itching
  Tonic—Maidenhair
  Wash—Ro. Chamomile, Rosemary
  Destroys Lice and Nits—Tincture of Larkspur
  Dye—Henna
  Prevent falling out—Oak, Maidenhair
  Keep Curl—Maidenhair
  Dressing—Bayberry
  Prevent premature baldness—Maidenhair

HANDS—see Chilblains, Tetters, Gout, Limbs
  Cold from sluggish circulation—Prickly Ash, Cayenne
  Scabs on children's—Spearmint
  Fissures (a split)—White Oak

HAYFEVER—A catarrhal affection of the mucous membrane of the eyes and respiratory tract due to the action of the pollen of certain plants.
  see Eyes, Respiratory tract
  Useful—Mullein

HEAD—CEPHALIC—pertaining to the Head
  See Headache, Brain
  Ringworm—Poke, paint on some Iodine
  Cold—Sanicle, Vinegar
  Nervine for Cranial pain—Lady's Slipper

Cranial neuralgia—Skullcap
Scald Head—Sanicle
Useful—Sage

HEADACHE—*see* Bilious, Indigestion, Constipation, Head, Migraine
Nervous—Vervain, Lady's Slipper, Catnip, Skullcap, Peppermint, Thyme
Sick—Vervain, Lobelia
Bilious—Roman Chamomile
Useful—Peppermint, Blessed Thistle, Coffee
Pain in back of head and base of brain—Black Cohosh

HEART (Cardiac)—*see* Arteries, Pulse, Chest, Blood, Hypertension
Palpitation—Motherwort, Tansy, Cayenne
Palpitation when chlorotic—Motherwort
Angina Pectoris—Ginger
Reduce pulse—Wild Cherry, Amer. Mandrake
Reduce heart action—Wild Cherry
Stimulant—Bitter Rt.
Sustains heart—Myrrh
Sustains heart before anaesthesia—Myrrh
Tonic—Motherwort, Amer. Centaury
Tonic to right or venous side—Golden Seal, Eur. Gentian
Heart's impulse becomes stronger and fuller—Serpentaria
Most powerful and persistent heart stimulant known—Cayenne
Acute palpitation—Cayenne
Pain—Sassafras
Strengthens—Blessed Thistle
Relieves heart by promoting outward circulation—Pleurisy Rt.
Useful—Cayenne, Motherwort, Coffee
Spasms—Sassafras
Weak—Motherwort

HEAT—*see* Exhaustion, Sunstroke
Prickly heat—take Vit. C
Specific for overheat—Pennyroyal

HEMORRHAGE—A discharge of blood, as from a ruptured blood vessel: profuse bleeding.

see Metorrhagia, Blood, Dysentery, Parturition, see organs involved

Useful—Hemlock Spruce, Yarrow, Bayberry, Comfrey, Purple Loosestrife, Witch Hazel, Catechu, Beth Rt., Cranesbill, False Unicorn

External and Internal—Oak, Cranesbill, Bistort

Intestinal—Sumach

Kidneys—Beth Rt.

Lungs (Pulmonary-Respiratory)—Cranesbill, Sumach, Beth Rt., Cayenne, Ginger, Bayberry, Mullein

Miscarriage threatened—False Unicorn

With debility—Peruvian Bark

Nose—Cranesbill

Passive—Peruvian Bark, Purple Loosestrife

Piles—Yarrow

Pregnancy—False Unicorn

Rectal—Butternut, Sumach, Witch Hazel

Urinary organs—Marshmallow

Uterine (Metorrhagia)—Mistletoe, Cranesbill, Sumach, Beth Rt., False Unicorn, Bayberry

HEMORRHOIDS (Piles)—A swelling formed by the dilation of a blood vessel at the anus.

see Anus, Rectum

Painful—Hemlock Spruce

Piles—Cascara Sagrada, Witch Hazel, Plantain, Figwort, Yarrow, Mullein, Poke

Bleeding piles—Witch Hazel

Stops hemorrhage in piles—Yarrow

Internal—Hemlock Spruce

Protrude—Hemlock Spruce, Yarrow

Useful—Butternut, Oak, Senna, Witch Hazel, Cascara Sagrada

Irritation and itching stopped—Balmony, Witch Hazel

HEPATIC—Pertaining to the liver

see Liver, Hepatitis, Jaundice, Fever, Gall Bladder

Useful—Aloes, Wahoo, Purple Loosestrife, Butternut, Bitter Rt., Polypody

Alterative—Yellow Parilla
Congestion—Wild Yam
Dropsy in chronic hepatic torpor—Balmony
Derangement—Dandelion
Derangement in Cholera—Purple Loosestrife
Gentle laxative—Polypody
Failure—Culver's Rt.
Hepatization (thickening of lung tissue)—Mullein
Tonic—White Poplar, Vervain, Culvers Rt., Red Raspberry, Oregon Grape
Torpor in eruptive diseases—Wahoo
Skin eruptions from congestions—Wahoo

HEPATITIS—Inflammation of the Liver
see Hepatic, Liver
Useful—Lobelia
Chronic—W. Horehound, Dandelion

HERNIA—see rupture

HICCOUGH—Often from acidity of the stomach
Try sticking out your tongue as far as you can, holding it with your teeth as long as possible; this often stops simple hiccoughs.

HOARSENESS—see Cold, Voice, Throat
Useful—Hyssop, Black and White Horehound, Licorice, Coltsfoot, Bayberry, Maidenhair, Marshmallow, Horseradish

HYDROPHOBIA—Canine madness; rabies, esp. in man.
Useful—Bitter Rt.

HYSTERIA—State of excessive irritability and feebleness of the nerves; morbid or senseless emotionalism.—see Nerves
Coughs—Lobeila
With debility—Peruvian Bark
With convulsions—Ladies Slipper, Black Cohosh, Asafoetida
In menstrual obstruction—Peppermint
Useful—Pennyroyal, Blue and Black Cohosh, G Rue, Hops, Lobelia, Motherwort, Spearmint, Asafoetida, Mistletoe, Valerian, Skullcap, Tansy, Catnip, Ladies Slipper, White Poplar, Peruvian Bark, Eur. Gentian, Skunk Cabbage

189

IMPETIGO—A skin disease marked by small pustules.
> *see* Eruptions, Tetters
Useful—Plantain

IMPOTENT—Wholly lacking in sexual power.
> *see* Barrenness, Sex, Generative Organs, Pregnancy
Relieved by True and False Unicorn Rt.

INDIGESTION—Incapability or difficulty in digesting food
> *see* Dyspepsia, Digestion, Digestive Organs, Headache
Atonic—Yellow Parilla, Myrrh
Atonic, relieve fermentation—Myrrh
Useful—Boneset, Ro. Chamomile, White Poplar, Motherwort, Pleurisy Rt., Ground Ivy, Dandelion, Cod Liver Oil
Relieves in lax condition of stomach—White Poplar

INFANTS' and CHILDREN'S TROUBLES—*see* Whooping Cough, Snuffles, Cholera, Thrush, Fever
Bed-wetting—*see* Urine
Bowel troubles—White Pond Lily, Red Elm, Rhubarb, Senna
Canker in stomach—Rue
Catarrh—Asafoetida
Colds—W. Horehound
Colic—Catnip
Coughs—Lobelia, Asafoetida, W. Horehound
Coughs, Whooping specific—Thyme
Cough and bronchitis, suffocating by phlegm—Lobelia
Food—Red Elm
Digestion weak—Rhubarb, Cod Liver Oil
Irritation of the alimentary canal—Rhubarb
Malnutrition—Olive Oil, Chickweed, Cod Liver Oil
Nerves—Ladies Slipper, Pennyroyal, Asafoetida, Valerian, Catnip
Purging—*see* Aloes
Stomach—Rhubarb, Raspberry, Peppermint
Scabs on hands and heads—Spearmint
Throat and mouth—Myrrh
Rickets—Olive Oil
Weaning of infants—Red Elm
Useful—Peppermint, Spearmint
Tonic—Rhubarb

Spasms—Skullcap
Restlessness in measles—Valerian
Restlessness in sleep—Catnip, Valerian

INFLAMMATIONS—A morbid condition of some part of the
   body, *see* Organs involved, Fevers
   Most obstinate—Marshmallow
   Internal—Chickweed, Red Elm, Linseed
   Useful—Hemlock Spruce, Chickweed, Hops, Linseed, Sassa-
      fras, Red Elm, Cayenne, Peppermint, Lobelia, Plantain,
      Wood Sage, Pleurisy Rt., Marshmallow, Figwort, White
      Pond Lily, Peruvian Bark, Cubebs

INFLUENZA—*see* Grippe

INTESTINAL—The lower part of the alimentary canal, extend-
      ing from the pylorus to the anus.
      see Digestive Organs, Alimentary Canal, Alvine Canal
   Catarrh—Horseradish
   Inflammation (Enteritis)—Red Elm
   Irritated—Red Elm, Wild Yam
   Irritated intestinal membrane—Linseed
   Intestinal indigestion—Motherwort
   Hemorrhage—Sumach
   False membrane removed—Yarrow
   Intestinal mucous membrane cleansed and toned—Linseed
   Large intestines stimulated—Aloes
   Tonic—Golden Seal
   Pylorus, inflamed or ulcerated—Red Elm
   Small intestines—Yellow Parilla, Culvers Rt.
   Stimulant—Bl. Pepper
   Worms expelled—American Wormseed
   Offensive odors—Charcoal

ITCHING—*see* Pruritus, Psora, Genital organs, Skin
   In eruptive diseases—Golden Seal
   Around genitals—Chickweed
   Measles—Golden Seal
   In smallpox—Golden Seal
   Caused by vermin in the hair—Tincture of Larkspur
   Useful—Burdock
   Piles—Witch Hazel

191

JAUNDICE—A morbid bodily condition due to the presence of
  bile-pigments in the blood, characterized by the yellow-
  ness of the skin; in rare instances by yellow vision.
    see Hepatic, Liver, Bile, Skin, Yellow Fever
  Useful—Culvers Rt., Barberry, Horseradish, Balmony, W.
    Horehound, Dandelion, Parsley, Yarrow, Amer. Mandrake,
    Bitter Rt., Hops, Lobelia, Wahoo
  Of extreme value—Eur. Gentian
  Acute—Boneset
  Bile absorbed tinging skin—Barberry
  Gall solidified—Culvers Rt.
  Chronic—Boneset, Balmony
  From occlusion—Bitter Rt.
  Overflow not from gall stones—Senna
  Pulse below par—Cayenne

JOINTS—see Rheumatism, Gout, Arthritis, Limbs, Bones
  Swollen—Mullein
  Stiffness—Mullein
  Painful—Mullein

KIDNEYS—see Albuminaria, Urine, Dysuria, Bright's Disease,
    Gravel, Bladder, Back, Stones
  Aching—Uva Ursi
  Atony—False Unicorn
  Catarrh—White Poplar
  Congested—Serpentaria, Parsley, Juniper, W. Poplar, Uva
    Ursi
  Dropsy tonic—Parsley, Pipsissewa
  Debility (weakness)—Tansy
  Dropsy—Parsley, Pipsissewa
  Inflammation (Nephritis)—Spearmint, Corn Silk
  Inflammation chronic—Uva Ursi
  Irritation—Gravel Rt., Marshmallow, Irish Moss
  Hemorrhages—Beth Root
  Mucous membrane—Bitter Rt., Ground Ivy
  Soothes—Corn Silk, Gravel Rt.
  Remove offensive odor—Charcoal
  Specific—Burdock
  Strengthens—Blessed Thistle, Purple Loosestrife
  Stone (Calculus-Gravel)—Parsley, Clivers, Gravel Rt.

Mucus in—Burdock

Tonic—Golden Seal, Balmony, Cranesbill, W. Poplar, Figwort

Torpor—Serpentaria, Juniper

Ulcerated—Uva Ursi, Comfrey

Urine, increase flow—*see* Urine

Useful—Hollyhock, Serpentaria, Black Cohosh, Burdock, Juniper, Plantain, Clivers, Hyssop, Horseradish, Gravel Rt., Maidenhair, Pipsissewa, Purple Loosestrife, Ground Ivy, Amer. Mandrake

LARYNGITIS—Inflammation of the larynx.
   see Voice
   Gargle—Vinegar, Sage
   Useful—Marshmallow

LEPROSY—Various loathsome skin diseases: (Hansen's disease).
   Useful—Burdock
   Eruptions—Red Elm
   Specific—Chaulmoogra, Calotropia

LEUCORRHOEA—A whitish mucous discharge from the Female Genital Organs—(Whites)
   see Vagina, Generative Organs
   Degenerate or foul—Amer. Columbo
   Lingering—Buchu
   Useful—Amer. Columbo, Yarrow, Uva Ursi, False Unicorn, Pipsissewa, Iceland Moss, Cranesbill, Witch Hazel, Golden Seal, Sumach, Red Raspberry, Sanicle, Beth Rt., White Poplar, Cubebs, Red Elm, Blue Cohosh, Purple Loosestrife, W. Oak, Catechu, Bistort, Hemlock Spruce, Bayberry, White Pond Lily, Pomegranate, Blue Flag

LIMBS—*see* Sciatica, Rheumatism, Joints, Bones, Palsy, Cramps, St. Vitus Dance, Hands, Feet
   Cramps in pregnancy—Cramp Bark
   Dropsied—Mullein
   Sore legs—White Pond Lily, Myrrh
   Dislocations, Sprains—Lobelia

LIVER—*see* Hepatic, Stones, Fever, Gall Bladder, Jaundice, Portal System, Bile, Blood impurities

Cholagogue—Eur. Gentian

Constipation—Boneset, Wahoo

Congested (engorged with blood)—Culvers Rt., Amer. Mandrake, Dandelion, Senna, Butternut

Cough with torpid liver—Wahoo

Dropsy in chronic hepatic torpor—Balmony

Chronic—Blue Flag, Oregon Grape Rt.

Inactive causing bilious fever—Culvers Rt.

Inactive in Typhoid, Typhus, Remitting, Rheumatic fevers and others—Culvers Rt.

Excreting tonic—Golden Seal, Dandelion, Wahoo, Culvers Rt.

Hard—W. Horehound

Inflammation—*see* Hepatitis

Mercury—Amer. Mandrake

Relaxant—Culvers Rt.

Secreting tonic—Golden Seal, Dandelion, Wahoo, Culvers Rt., Boneset

Tubuli—Bitter Rt.

Skin diseases of hepatic origin—Wahoo

Stimulating—Coffee

Stimulating to the Liver Tubuli—Culvers Rt.

Secretions corrected—Barberry

Strengthens—Blessed Thistle

Tonic—Amer. Centaury, Wahoo, Rhubarb, Boneset, Oregon Grape

Tonic to portal circulation—Golden Seal

Torpor—Balmony, Horseradish, Boneset, Cascara Sagrada, Dandelion, Culvers Rt.

Obstructions—Dandelion

Useful—Blue Flag, Bitter Rt., Pipsissewa, Black Cohosh, Boneset, Hops, Lobelia, Yellow Parilla, Amer. Mandrake, Cascara Sagrada, Senna, Ground Ivy, Barberry, Hyssop, Blessed Thistle, Queen's Delight, Yarrow, Boneset, Purple Loosestrife

LOCHIA—Liquid discharge from the uterus after childbirth.
see Parturition
When scanty—Motherwort

LOCKJAW—Form of tetanus in which the jaws become locked firmly together.

LUMBAGO—MYALGIA in the lumbar region: pain in the
      muscles of the loins and the small of the back; muscular
      rheumatism.
      see Back, Rheumatism
   Aching—Plantain, Bayberry
   Useful—Juniper, Parsley, Poke

LUNGS—*see* Pulmonary, Pleurisy, Pneumonia, Tuberculosis,
      Bronchitis, Chest, Phthisis, Respiratory Organs, Breath,
      Colds, Coughs, Hemorrhage
   Air passages cleaned—Lobelia
   Bleeding—Red Elm, Chickweed
   Congestion—W. Horehound
   Cleansing—Elecampane, Lobelia
   Chronic—W. Horehound, Elecampane
   Excessive expectoration—W. Horehound, Elecampane
   Emphysema (malfunction of air sacs)—Cheken
   Fever (lung), where skin is hot and pulse rigid—Pleurisy Rt.
   Hyperaemic conditions—W. Horehound
   Hepatization or thickening of lung tissue—Mullein
   Inflammation—Comfrey, Chickweed, Red Elm
   Phlegm loosened—W. Horehound, Elecampane
   Specific—Pleurisy Rt.
   Snuff—Wild Cherry
   Mucous membrane—Iceland Moss, Linseed
   Tonic—Pleurisy Rt., Comfrey, Elecampane, Myrrh, Blessed
      Thistle
   Ulcerated—Comfrey, Sanicle
   Useful—Lobelia, Hyssop, Yellow Parilla, White and Black
      Horehound, Thyme, Pleurisy Rt., Licorice, Coltsfoot, Wild
      Cherry, Black Cohosh, Ro. Chamomile

LYMPHATICS—Vessels containing or conveying lymph.
      see Glands, Scrofula
   Debility—Blue Flag
   Inflammatory swelling in groins—see Buboes
   Veins varicosed—Witch Hazel
   Useful—Black Cohosh, Blue Flag, Pipsissewa, Burdock,
      Prickly Ash

MALARIA—A febrile disease, usually intermittent or remittent,
      and characterized by attacks of chills, fever, sweating.

Formerly supposed to be due to swamp exhalations but now believed to be caused by parasitic protozoans which are transferred to the human blood by mosquitoes and which occupy and destroy the red blood corpuscles.

see Miasma, Ague, Intermittent and remittent fevers

To get rid of malaria in swamp regions—Plant Eucalyptus and Sunflowers

MEASLES—Acute infectious disease occurring mostly in children, characterized by catarrhal and febrile symptoms and an eruption of small red spots: RUBEOLA: also RUBELLA (German Measles).

see Eruptions

When eruputions are slow—Yarrow

Fever—Sanicle

Itching and burning skin—Golden Seal

Specific—Pleurisy Rt.

Restless Children—Valerian

During scaling process—Red Elm

Useful—Peppermint, Yarrow, Hyssop, Asafoetida, Peruvian Bark

MELANCHOLY—Gloomy state of mind: depression, sadness.

see Mind

Useful—Thyme

MENINGES—Spinal Meningitis—Spotted Fever—Inflammation of the meninges.

see Phrenitis

Cerebro-spinal—Boneset

Useful—Asafoetida, Boneset, Lobelia

MENNORRHAGIA—Excessive menstrual discharge

Useful—Black Horehound, Beth Rt., Bayberry, True and False Unicorn, Cranesbill, Pennyroyal

MENSTRUATION—Monthly discharge of blood from the uterus, occuring in women

see Amenorrhea, Dysmenorrhoea, Mennorrhagia

Assist flow during puerperal convulsions—Blue Chohosh

Promotes flow (Emmenagogue)—Motherwort, Ro. Chamomile, Amer. Centaury, Pleurisy Rt., Blue Cohosh, Wild Yam

Induces flow after parturition—Blue Cohosh
Hysteria in obstruction—Peppermint
Obstructed—Peppermint, Parsley, Wood Sage
Painful—White Poplar, Cramp Bark, Tansy
Irregular—Figwort
Suppressed from cold—*see* Amenorrhea
Aching back and pelvis in tardy menstruction—Motherwort
Useful—Catnip, Wild Yam, Myrrh
Congested—Ginger
Tardy—Foot bath with Mustard or Cayenne

MERCURY—Quicksilver, a preparation of which is used in medicine.
see Debility
Mercurial sore mouth—Sumach
Salivation—Cranesbill, Sumach
Rheumatism—Yellow Parilla
Superior for Liver—Amer. Mandrake
Cachexia—Bayberry, Blue Flag, Guaiacum

METRORRHAGIA—Excessive discharge of blood from the uterus, esp. when not menstrual. *See* Hemorrhage

MIASMA—Noxious exhalations from putrescent organic matter, poisonous effluvis, or germs infecting the atmosphere. *See* Malaria
Neutralizes malarious regions—Sunflower, Eucalyptus

MICTURITION—Morbidly frequent urination.
see Urine, Stranguria, Dysuria

MIGRAINE (Hemicrania)—A kind of severe headache, limited usually to one side of the head, and often accompanied by nausea.
see Headache
Useful—Peruvian Bark, Valerian, Blessed Thistle

MILK—*see* Breast, Parturition
Promotes—Goat's Rue, Red Raspberry
Resembles breast milk—add Papaya to regular milk
Stop flow of milk—Sage
Prevent milk from forming—Sage

Produces free supply of milk—Marshmallow
Enriches milk in nursing mothers—Marshmallow

MIND—Memory, thought, remembrance.
    see Melancholy
    Clear—Coffee

MISCARRIAGE—Premature expulsion of a fetus from the uterus,
    esp., before it is viable.
    see Pregnancy, Back
    To prevent—Cramp Bark, Beth Rt., False and True Unicorn,
      Wild Yam
    To stop hemorrhage in threatened—False Unicorn
    Tonic—Amer. Columbo
    After-pain and hemorrhage—False Unicorn

MOLES—*See* Growths

MOUTH—*see* Fauces
    Aphthous sore (ulcers due to parasitic fungus in mouth and
      intestinal canal; esp. thrush)—Amer. Columbo, White
      Pond Lily, Myrrh, Sumach
    Canker—Red Raspberry
    Infant's spray—Myrrh
    Irritated—White Pond Lily
    Mercurical—Sumach
    Increases flow of saliva—*see* Saliva
    Sores—Hemlock Spruce, Cranesbill, Witch Hazel, Golden
      Seal, Bistort, White Oak
    Ulcerated—Sage, Myrrh, Sanicle, Bistort, Golden Seal, Pom-
      egranate
    White (Frog)—*see* Thrush
    Wash—Peruvian Bark, Golden Seal, Barberry

MUCUS and MUCOUS MEMBRANES
    see Catarrh, Croup, Diphtheria, Phlegm, Gastritis, Expec-
      toration, and organs involved
    Aged, debilitated conditions—Hyssop
    Cleansing accumulated mucus in catarrh and irritated con-
      ditions as in—
    Alvine Tract—Culvers Rt., Queen's Delight, Wild Cherry,
      Senna, Eur. and Amer. Columbo, Aloes, Elecampane, Lin-
      seed, Rhubarb, Oregon Grape, Cranesbill

Alvine tonic—Butternut
Bloody mucous—Iceland Moss
Canker—Red Raspberry
Cystic (Bladder)—Corn Silk
Babies—*see* Snuffles
Debilitated conditions—Golden Seal, Hyssop, Guaiacum
Dry—Prickly Ash
Excessive mucous discharge—Catechu
Gastric—Elecampane, Wahoo
Generative (Genital) Organs—Beth Rt., Uva Ursi
Irritation and inflammation—Marshmallow
Mucus abundant, not easily expectorated—Myrrh
Mucus, cast off accumulated—Pipsissewa, Hyssop
Tonic—False Unicorn, Red Raspberry, Bl. Horehound
Urinary—Gravel Rt., Uva Ursi, Cubebs, Plantain, Linseed
Useful for all mucous membranes—Golden Seal, White Pond
  Lily, Prickly Ash, White Poplar, Uva Ursi, Beth Rt., Yellow
  Parilla, Maiden Hair, Yarrow, Hollyhock, Mullein, Purple
  Loosestrife, Red Raspberry, Amer. Mandrake, Horse-
  radish, Witch Hazel, Elecampane, Poke, Plantain, Wahoo,
  Ground Ivy, Roman Chamomile, Wild Cherry, Red Elm,
  Marshmallow, Pleurisy Rt., Lobelia, Amer. and Eur. Co-
  lumbo, Coltsfoot, Rhubarb, Bayberry

MUMPS—Infectious disease characterized by inflammatory swelling of the paratoid and (usually) other salivary glands,
  and sometimes inflammation of the testicles, ovaries, etc.
  see Face, Glands, Saliva
  Useful—Mullein

MUSCLES—*see* Rheumatism, Palsy, Chorea
  Muscular Membrane of Bowels—Bitter Rt.
  Dislocations—Lobelia
  Relaxant—Lobelia
  Relaxant to muscle fibre—Blue Cohosh, Wild Yam
  Rigidity—*see* Palsy
  Strengthens—Purple Loosestrife, Sage
  Tonic—Tansy
  Weakness—*see* Palsy
  Weakness causing Nocturnal incontinence—*see* Enuresis
  Palsy—Tansy

NAUSEA—Sickness at the stomach—sensation of impending vomiting—*see* Vomiting, Bilious, Charcoal, Pregnancy
Useful—Ginger, Cloves, Spearmint, Red Raspberry, Peppermint, Pennyroyal, Wild Yam, Sage

NECK—*see* Cervix, Lymphatics, Thyroid
Hardened—*see* Goitre

NERVES—*see* Convalescence, Delirium, St. Vitus Dance, Bilious,
Infants, Back and Organs involved, Constipation, Convulsions, Fever, Hysteria, Sleep, Headache, Sciatica
Auditory tension—too much Quinine or Peruvian Bark
Cerebral—Peruvian Bark, Skullcap, Sage, Mistletoe
Central—Lobelia, Peruvian Bark
Debilitated, weak, enfeebled conditions—Valerian, Lady's
Slipper, Asafoetida, Mistletoe
Excitement—Black Cohosh, Wild Yam
Exhaustion (Neurasthenia) and depression—Hops
Gonorrhea—Clivers
Relieved, Irritated—Valerian, Lady's Slipper, Asafoetida,
Blue Cohosh, Motherwort, Wild Cherry, True Unicorn,
Clivers
Irritated during Parturition—Blue Cohosh, Lady's Slipper,
Myrrh
Irritated in dysmenorrhea—Roman Chamomile, Pennyroyal
Irritated nervous depression—Lady's Slipper, True Unicorn
Hypochondria (fancied ill health)—Asafoetida, Skullcap,
Valerian
Nutritious—Oats
Peripheral—Peruvian Bark
Nervous prostration—Skullcap, Yarrow
Sympathetic system—Lobelia, Peruvian Bark, Skullcap
Spinal—Lobelia, Peruvian Bark, Skullcap, Golden Seal
Steady after anaesthesia—Myrrh
Tremors—Hops
Tonic—Amer. Centaury, Myrrh, Valerian, Skullcap, Gravel
Rt., Peruvian Bk.
Useful—Ro. Chamomile, Black and Blue Cohosh, Ground Ivy
Lady's Slipper, Asafoetida, Skullcap, Catnip, Peruvian Bark,
Hops, Lobelia, Red Raspberry, Valerian, Coffee, Mistletoe, Red Clover, Tansy, Red Elm, Vervain, Sage, Bur-

dock, Purple Loosestrife, Wild Yam, Serpentaria, Cayenne, Buchu, Skunk Cabbage, Thyme
Rheumatism—Wild Yam
Depression—Hops, Lady's Slipper

NEURALGIA—Pain, usually sharp and paroxysmal, along the course of a nerve.
 see Nerves, Sciatica
Chronic—Prickly Ash
Cranial—Skullcap
Facial—Skullcap, Wild Yam
Swellings—Sassafras
Useful—Cayenne, Horseradish, Lady's Slipper, Cramp Bark, Peruvian Bark, Hops, Poke, Marshmallow, Valerian, Blue Cohosh, Peppermint, Ro. Chamomile

NIPPLES—Mamilla—*see* Breast

NOSE—*see* Cold, Snuffles
Hemorrhage—Craneshill
Bleeding (EPISTAXIS)—Witch Hazel
Catarrh—Skunk Cabbage, Mullein, Bayberry, Spearmint, Comfrey, Witch Hazel, Golden Seal
Congestions—Golden Seal, Cubebs, Comfrey, Mullein, Maidenhair, Bayberry
Mucous membrane—Spearmint
Mucous membrane, acute inflammation (Coryza)—Inhale steam of Hyssop

OPHTHALMIA—Inflammation of the eye, esp. of its membrane structures—both external and internal.
 see Eye
Catarrhal—Cranesbill
Grandular with Ulceration of the Cornea, Golden Seal
Purulent—White Poplar, Witch Hazel
Purulent with pus—White Pond Lily, Red Elm
Useful—Marshmallow, Burdock, Golden Seal, Lobelia, Plantain, Red Raspberry, Mullein, White Pond Lily, White Poplar

OPIUM—Poppy (PAPAVER SOMNIFERUM) juice, containing morphine

Resists stupefying influence—Coffee
Replace—Hops
Useful—Skullcap

OVARIES—*see* Generative Organs
Inflammation (OVARITIS)—Red Elm, *see* Mumps
Tonic—False Unicorn
Best relaxant—Cramp Bark

PAINS—*see* Organ affected
Useful—Black Cohosh, Valerian, Hops, Spearmint, Lobelia,
Wild Yam, Peruvian Bark, Buchu, Marshmallow
In the Sacral region—Yarrow

PALATE—Roof of the mouth—*see* Uvula

PALSY—Paralysis, esp. progressive form
see Paralysis, Limbs, Muscular
Useful—Horseradish, Sage, Tansy, Cayenne

PARALYSIS—Impairment or loss of power of voluntary motion or
of sensation. *see* Palsy
Fauces—Ginger
Tongue—Ginger
Useful—Prickly Ash, Cayenne

PARTURITION—(Childbirth)
see Lochia, Pregnancy, Uterus, Milk
Expedite—Blue Cohosh
Circulation equalized—Myrrh, Serpentaria
Extremities cold—Serpentaria
Delivery easy and speedy—Red Raspberry
Excellent—Myrrh, Black Cohosh, Beth Root
Contractions firmer—Bayberry
Contractions stimulated—Mistletoe, Blue Cohosh
Contractions sustained—Myrrh
Hemorrhagic tendency—Myrrh, Beth Rt., Mistletoe, Bay-
berry, Red Raspberry, Serpentaria
Irritation of the nerves—Blue Cohosh, Lady's Slipper, Myrrh
Nerves quieted—Wild Yam, Blue Cohosh
Induce menstruation after—Blue and Black Cohosh
Pains inefficient—Serpentaria, Mistletoe
Post-partem hemorrhage—Lady's Slipper

Preparatory—True Unicorn, Wild Yam, Beth Rt.
Puerperal Septicaemia (blood poisoning)—Echinacea
Puerperal Convulsions—Blue and Black Cohosh, Skullcap,
    Lobelia
Assist in relieving flow during convulsions—Blue Cohosh
Assists expulsion of placenta when retained—Mistletoe
After-pains—Blue Cohosh, Ladys' Slipper, Motherwort, Wild
    Yam, Red Raspberry
To umbilicus, after removing cord—Myrrh
Relieves rigid os uteri (orifice of the Uterus)—Lady's Slipper

PELVIS
Aching in tardy menstruation—Motherwort
Aching in hips—Buchu
Congestion—Buchu
Nerves—Buchu, Asafoetida
Tonic—Gravel Rt., Uva Ursi, Figwort
Tonic to mucous membrane of Pelvic Canal—Wild Cherry
Weakness—Gravel Rt., Blessed Thistle
Useful—Black Cohosh, Amer. Mandrake

PENICILLIN—
An old remedy—Scrape green mould off stale bread; 1 tea-
    spoon mould to 1 cup water.

PENIS—*see* Prepuce
Discharges and aching—Buchu

PERIOSTEAL—PERIOSTITIS—Inflammation of the periosteum,
the dense fibrous membrane covering the surface of the
bones except at their cartilaginous extremities.
see Inflammation, Bones
Useful—Mullein

PERITONITIS—Inflammation of the peritoneum, the serous mem-
brane lining the abdominal cavity.
see Serous membrane, Ascitis
Useful—Pleurisy Rt., Mullein, Lobelia, Chickweed

PERSPIRATION (Sweats)
Hectic fever—Sage
Scrofula—Poke
Glands—Pleurisy Rt.

Exhaustive in hectic fevers—Sage, Pomegranate
Cold and clammy—Cayenne
Obstructed—Yarrow
Feet—White Oak
Produce—Yarrow, Spearmint, Black Pepper, Catnip, Thistle
Night sweats relieved—Yarrow
Night sweats relieved in Phthisis—Boneset, Pomegranate
Fetid—White Poplar

PHARYNGITIS—Inflammation of the mucous membrane of the
  Pharynx
  see Fauces
  Irritated and inflamed—White Pond Lily, Red Elm, Marshmallow

PHLEGM—The thick mucus secreted in the respiratory passages
  and discharged by coughing, etc.
  see Mucus, Expectoration
  Loosens—W. Horehound, Lobelia, Elecampane
  Obstructed by—Lobelia
  Suffocating from—Lobelia

PHRENITIS—Inflammation of the brain or its meninges, attended
  with fever and delirium
  Useful—Lobelia, Asafoetida

PHTHISIS—A wasting away, esp. tuberculosis of the lungs.
  see Catarrh, Respiratory organs
  Night sweats—Boneset, Pomegranate, Myrrh
  Hectic fever—Eur. Columbo
  Useful—Yarrow, W. Horehound, Mullein, Yellow Parilla
  Phthisis Pulmonalis—Myrrh
  Expectoration too free—Ground Ivy
  see Blood purifiers—Pipsissewa

PIMPLE—(Papule) usually inflammatory but not suppurative
  see Eruption
  Useful—Burdock

PLEURITIS—PLEURISY—Inflammation of the pleura, a delicate
  serous membrane investing each lung.
  see Pneumonia, Respiratory organs, Chest
  Difficult breathing—Pleurisy Rt.

Most valuable—Pleurisy Rt., Lobelia, Mullein
Effusions—Mullein
Useful—Cayenne, Pleurisy Rt., Skunk Cabbage

PNEUMONIA—Acute inflammation of the Lungs
    see Pleurisy, Respiratory Organs, Chest
With biliousness and constipation—Boneset
Lung poultice—Linseed
Useful—Irish Moss, Red Elm, Lobelia, Pleurisy Rt., Ginger,
    Linseed

POISONING—Any substance which tends to destroy life or impair health when taken into the system.
    see Bites, Coma, Septic
Antidote—Olive Oil, Boneset
Blood—Chickweed, Plantain, Echinacea
Cholaemic (Bile salts in the blood)—Wahoo
Lead or painters—Ground Ivy, Red Elm
Gas (World War I)—Lily of the Valley
Ivy—Echinacea, Paste of slaked lime
Narcotic—Coffee, Bayberry, Lobelia emetic
Narcotic substitute—Lobelia
Sumac—Serpentaria
Useful—G. Rue, Mullein
Sores—Lobelia

PORTAL SYSTEM—Pertaining to the portal vein, the large vein
    conveying blood to the liver from the veins of the stomach,
    intestine, and spleen.
    see Circulation, Liver
Relieves—Butternut
Tonic—Cayenne,, Golden Seal

PREGNANCY—*see* Parturition, Barrenness, Miscarriage
After-pains—Wild Yam
Complications—False Unicorn
Convalescence—Red Raspberry
Cramps—Cramp Bark
Cramps, limbs—Cramp Bark
Cramps, Uterine—Wild Yam
Dyspepsia relieved—True Unicorn
Hemorrhage in threatened miscarriage—False Unicorn

205

Impotency and barrenness relieved—True and False Unicorn
Nausea and vomiting—Eur. Columbo, Spearmint, Wild Yam,
Cloves, Golden Seal, Myrrh
Nervous—Wild Yam, Cramp Bark
Pains (false) and restlessness—Blue Cohosh
Irritation and pains—Wild Yam
Hemorrhage—False Unicorn
Stomach troubles—False and True Unicorn
Tonic, Gastric—False Unicorn
Delivery prompt and easy—False Unicorn, Red Raspberry
Tonic, Uterine—False Unicorn
Useful—True and False Unicorn, Red Raspberry, Wild Yam,
Eur. Columbo
To umbilicus, after removing cord—Myrrh

PREPUCE—The foreskin—*see* Penis, Chancre
Irritable chancres and excoriations—White Pond Lily

PROSTATE—Large gland surrounding the commencement of
the male urethra in front of the mouth of the bladder.
see Glands
Congestion with discharges and aching of penis—Buchu
Prostatitis (irritated and inflamed)—White Pond Lily,
Gravel Rt.
Useful—Gravel Rt., Buchu, Hollyhock
Weakness—Uva Ursi

PRURITUS—Itching, esp., when without visible eruption; se-
vere irritation and inflammation of the skin.
see Itching, Skin
Pruritis Ani—*see* Anus
Pruritis Vulva—Tansy
Useful—Hops, Peppermint, Red Elm

PSORA—Itch from the Itch-mite
Useful—Elecampane, Poke

PSORIASIS—Chronic skin disease characterized by formation of
scaly patches.
see Eruptions Scrofula, Skin, Cutaneous
Useful—Chaumoogra, Olive Oil

PULMONARY TROUBLES—Affecting the lungs

see Tuberculosis, Colds, Respiratory organs, Hemorrhage
Useful—Iceland Moss, Mullein, Maidenhair, Sanicle, Ground
    Ivy, Amer. Mandrake, Eur. Columbo, Thyme
Catarrh—Pleurisy Rt.
Debilitated—Coltsfoot, Balm of Gilead
Mucous membrane—Elecampane
Tobacco—Coltsfoot
Acute and chronic—Marshmallow

PULSE—*see* Arteries, Heart
Lessens frequency—Wild Cherry, Amer. Mandrake
Rigid in fevers—Pleurisy Rt.
Rigid in Rheumatic fever—Pleurisy Rt.
Below par in jaundice—Cayenne
Stenic (morbid increase of vital or cardiac action)—Pleurisy
    Rt.
In rheumatism—Black Cohosh
Increases pulse in acute and chronic rheumatism—Black
    Cohosh
Produces fullness—Horse Radish, Black Cohosh
Fuller and better before anaesthesia—Myrrh
Reduce in tuberculosis—Black Cohosh

PUS—A yellowish-white, more or less viscid substance consisting
    of a liquid plasma in which leucocytes, etc. are suspended.
Excessive reduced—Poke Peruvian Bark
Useful—Peruvian Bark, Comfrey

PUTREFACTION—Rotting; decomposition.
    see Septic
Removes and arrests foul odors—Myrrh, Lobelia, Charcoal
Foul sore in throat—White Pond Lily, Bayberry, Pineapple
Ulcers—Carrot
With nerve irritation—Lady's Slipper
Dislodge semi-putrescent material—Lobelia

PYLORUS—Opening between the stomach and intestine
    see stomach and intestine.
Inflammation or ulceration—Red Elm

QUININE
Tonic substitute—White Poplar

Better than—Skullcap
Substitute—Parsley, Senna
Alcoholics cannot take—Black Pepper
In excess—Peruvian Bark

QUINSY—Suppurative inflammation of the tonsils: suppurative
tonsilitis. *See* Tonsils, Throat
Gargle—Sanicle, Sage, Purple Loosestrife, Cayenne
Neck compress—Cayenne
Infusion—Cayenne

RECTUM—*see* Anus, Hemorrhoids, Colitis
To cool—Cubebs
Fissures (a split)—White Oak
Hemorrhages—Butternut, Sumach, Witch Hazel
Irritation—Witch Hazel
Nutrition—Olive Oil fed through rectum
Prolapsus Ani (falling down of the rectum)—Witch Hazel,
Oak, Sumach, White Poplar
Ulcers—Hemlock Spruce
Weakness—White Poplar

RESPIRATORY ORGANS—Breathing organs
see Lungs, Bronchial, Pulmonary troubles, coughs, Expec-
toration, Pneumonia, Phthisis, Convulsions, Hemorrhage,
Breath, Asthma, Grippe, Pleurisy
Catarrh—Polypody Root, Black and White Horehound
Cold—Sanicle
Expectorate—Black Horehound
Expectorate mucous from irritated and inflamed membrane—
Linseed
Hayfever—Mullein
Tonic—Black and White Horehound, Comfrey, Golden Seal
Tonic to the Mucous membrane—Wild Cherry, Black Hore-
hound, Comfrey Rt., Hollyhock
Tonic to Mucous membrane of the respiratory tubuli—Ground
Ivy
Tubuli—Lobelia
Useful—Black Horehound, Balm of Gilead, Yellow Parilla,
Wild Cherry

RHEUMATIC FEVER—*see* Rheumatism, Fever
    Liver is not active enough—Culver's Rt.
    Skin hot, pulse rigid—Pleurisy Root
    Useful—Lobelia, Pleurisy Rt.

RHEUMATISM (Acute or inflammatory)—Characterized by inflammation of the joints, accompanied by constitutional disturbances; also any of various other diseases of the joints or muscles as chronic joint inflammations (chronic rheumatism) and certain painful affections of the muscles (muscular rheumatism).
    see Arthritis, Gout, Joints, Rheumatic fever, Lumbago, Muscles
    Acute—Poke, Black Cohosh, Buchu, Gravel Rt., Pleurisy Rt., Wood Sage
    Articular—Hops
        see Blood impurities—Pipsissewa, Jam Sarsaparilla
    Bilious—Boneset
    Chronic—Blue Flag, Poke, Sassafras, Black Cohosh, Buchu, Guaiacum, Skunk Cabbage, Prickly Ash, Jam Sarsaparilla
    Gouty—Boneset
    Inflammatory—Boneset
    Ligamentous (connecting tissue)—Poke
    Mercurial—Yellow Parilla
    Nervous—Wild Yam
    Scrofulous—Yellow Parilla
    Synovial (membrane covering joints)—Poke
    Useful—Hemlock Spruce, Burdock, Blue and Black Cohosh, Guaiacum, Blue Flag, Sassafras, Lobelia, Cayenne, Wahoo, Pipsissewa, Lady's Slipper, Dandelion, Poke, Boneset, Yellow Parilla, Chickweed, Pennyroyal, Mullein, Serpentaria, Juniper, Horseradish, Hops, Jam Sarsaparilla, Queen's Delight, Prickly Ash
    Uterine—Cramp Bark, Black Cohosh
    Venereal—Guaiacum

RICKETS—A disease of childhood, characterized by softening of the bones through perverted nutrition and often resulting in deformities.
    Infants—Olive Oil

Useful—Skullcap, Olive Oil

RINGWORM (HERPES SERPIGO)—Contagious skin disease
due to parasites and characterized by the formation of
ring-shaped eruptive patches.
see Skin, Eruptions
Useful—White Oak, Red Elm, Poke, Golden Seal
Paint with light covering of iodine
Scalp—Poke

RUPTURE (HERNIA)—esp. an abdominal break.
Strangulated—Lobelia

ST. VITUS DANCE—The disease chorea. *See* chorea, nerves

SALIVA—Fluid discharged by glands into the mouth to keep
the mouth moist and aid mastication and digestion.
see Mumps, Mouth, Glands
Mercurial salivation (abnormally abundant flow of saliva)
Yellow—Rhubarb
Stimulates salivary glands—Ginger, Prickly Ash, Blue Flag,
Balmony, Amer. Mandrake, Poke

SCARLATINA—A mild form of scarlet fever.
Scarlatina Malignans—Cayenne, Peruvian Bark
Excellent—Burdock
During scaling process—Red Elm
Prevent scales from being spread around the room—wash
with Golden Seal

SCARLET FEVER—A contagious febrile disease characterized
by a scarlet eruption.
see Fevers, Scarlatina, Eruptions
Restless children—Valerian
Malignant Scarlet Fever—Lobelia
Useful—Hyssop, Pleurisy Rt., Lobelia, Cayenne

SCIATICA—Inflammation of the sciatic nerve, sciatic neuralgia.
Useful—Juniper, Poke, Buchu, Wild Yam, Ground Ivy

SCROFULA or SCROFULOUS—A constitutional disorder of a tu-
berculous nature characterized chiefly by swelling and

degeneration of the lymphatic glands, esp. of the neck, and by inflammation of the joints, etc. (King's Evil)
see Tuberculosis, Lymphatics, Psoriasis
Chlorotic with scrofulous inpurity—Motherwort
Debility—Pipsissewa, Blue Flag, Peruvian Bark
see Blood purifiers, Queen's Delight, Jam. Sarsaparilla, Poke, Pipsissiwa, Black Cohosh, Motherwort
Hectic fever—Wild Cherry
Diarrhea and Dysentery—Plantain, Pipsissewa
Eyes—see Ophthalmia
Prevent—Bayberry
Rheumatism—Yellow Parilla
Saliva flow increased—see Saliva
Sores—White Pond Lily, Carrot, Coltsfoot
Swellings—Plantain, Mullein
Useful—Burdock, Pipsissewa, Black Cohosh, Blue Flag, Yellow Parilla, Poke, Plantain, Figwort, Jam Sarsaparilla, Queen's Delight, Oregon Grape, Peruvian Bark, Clivers, White Oak, Sanicle, Eur. Gentian, Sassafras, Guaiacum, Amer. Mandrake

SCURVY—(SCORBUTIC)—A disease characterized by swollen and bleeding gums, livid spots on the skin, due esp. to unvaried diet, esp. one without vegetables.
see Gums, Skin
Specific (anti-scorbutic)—Clivers, Sanicle
Useful—Juniper, Burdock, Queen's Delight, Pipsissewa, Horseradish, Sassafras

SEBACEOUS—Pertaining to glands, follicles, etc. which secrete oily matter for lubricating hair and skin. See Glands
Useful—Burdock

SECERNENT—Secretion as applied to function of a gland
Clogged—Guaiacum
Useful—Black Cohosh, Blue Flag, Hops, Yellow Parilla, Ground Ivy, Figwort, Pipsissewa

SEPTIC—Poisoning of the system due to the entrance of putrefactive material into the blood. See Putrefaction
Black tongue in low septic conditions—Echinacea

Puerperal septicaemia (blood poisoning)—Echinacea
Prevents—Myrrh

SEROUS—Resembling or containing serum—SEROUS FLUID—
any fluids resembling blood-serum as the fluids of the serous membranes. SEROUS MEMBRANE— any of the
various thin membranes, as the peritoneum, which line
certain cavities of the body and exude a serous fluid.
see Peritonitis
Membranes—Lobelia, Poke, Black Cohosh, Mullein, Prickly
Ash, Pleurisy Rt.

SEXUAL—*see* Spermatorrhea, Barrenness, Generative Organs
Excess desire—Hops
Uncontrollable desire in Women (Nymphomania) Lady's
Slipper, Hops
Impotency relieved—True and False Unicorn
Painful erections in Gonorrhea—Hops

SHINGLES (HERPES ZOSTER)—A cutaneous disease characterized by vesicles which sometimes form a girdle about
the body.
see Cutaneous, Tetters
Relieve burning pain—rub on Oil of Peppermint, Red Elm

SHOCK
Of injury—Cayenne, Myrrh

SKIN—*see* Cutaneous, Eczemas, Tetters, Psoriasis, Eruptions,
Bruises, Pruritus, Scurvy, Erysipelas
Abraded and denuded, excoriated surfaces—Red Elm, Marsh-
mallow, White Pond Lily
Chafy—Oregon Grape, White Pond Lily
Cold—Prickly Ash, Cayenne
Cold Cream—Rosewater, Almond Oil, and Attar of Roses
Contagious—Poke
Circulation (surface)—*see* Capillaries
Alterative—Yellow Parilla, Polypody, Sassafras
Hardened (Callous)—rub with Vaseline or Olive Oil
Diseases—Red Elm, Elecampane, Figwort, Blue Flag
Diseases of Hepatic origin—Wahoo
see Blood purifiers—Black Cohosh

Fishskin (ICHTHYOSIS)—Vit. A, Cod Liver Oil
Heat, excessive—Pleurisy Rt.
Heat, in Lung Fever—Pleurisy Rt.
Heat in Rheumatic Fever—Pleurisy Rt.
Irritation and inflammation—Plantain, Poke, Red Elm, Chick-
weed, Black Cohosh, Linseed
Measles, burning and itching—Golden Seal
Pigment lack (VITILIGO)—cover with walnut juice
Scaly—Witch Hazel, Red Clover, White Oak, Oregon Grape,
Red Elm
Sunburn—Aloes, wash with cucumbers
Smallpox, burning and itching—Golden Seal
Scabs on hands and heads—Spearmint
Scabies—Poke, Sassafras
Toadskin (PHRYNODERMA)—Vit. A, Cod Liver Oil
Tinged from absorbed bile—Barberry, see Jaundice
Useful—Burdock, Chickweed, Pipsissewa, Horseradish, Blue
Flag, Yellow Parilla, Wood Sage, Poke, Serpentaria,
Golden Seal, Aloes, Oregon Grape, Red Elm, Witch Hazel,
Clivers, Barberry, Ground Ivy, Queen's Delight, Yarrow,
Juniper, Loosestrife
Yellow (Jaundiced)—Barberry

SLEEP—see Nerves
Arterial excitement quieted—Yarrow
Children's restlessness—Catnip, Valerian
Cholera—Purple Loosestrife
Opium victim—Skullcap
Overwrought—Hops
Nerve irritation—Lady's Slipper
Restless relieved—Asafoetida, Hops, Skunk Cabbage, Penny-
royal, Skullcap, Valerian, Wild Yam
Restless relieved in low fever—Valerian
Restlessness relieved in insanity—Lady's Slipper
Sleeplessness (Insomnia)—Vervain, Valerian, Skullcap, Hops,
Motherwort, Lady's Slipper, Asafoetida, Thyme, Black
Cohosh, Catnip
Morbid—Hops, Valerian
Nightmare—Melancholy—Thyme

SMALLPOX—An acute, highly contagious febrile disease characterized by a pustular eruption which often leaves permanent pits or scars—(VARIOLA).

see Eruptions, Fever

Allays itching and burning—Golden Seal

Relieves nervous system—Golden Seal

Tones new cuticle under postules—Golden Seal, Sweet Oil

Useful—Golden Seal, Peruvian Bark, Black Cohosh

SNUFFLES—To draw the breath or mucous through the nostrils in a noisy manner because of mucous accumulations in the nose.

Apply equal parts hot milk and olive oil up nostrils with a camel hair brush 3 or 4 times daily

SORES

see Organs involved, Gangrene, Scrofula, Bruises, Canker

Festering (infected)—Marshmallow, Red Elm

Irritated—Butternut, Comfrey

Old—Prickly Ash

Poisoned—Lobelia

Rusty nail—Lobelia

Running—Sanicle

Useful—Clivers, Lobelia, White Oak, Figwort, Sassafrass, Red Elm, Carrot, Balm of Gilead, White Pond Lily, Ground Ivy, Purple Loosestrife, Plantain, Hops, Chickweed, Myrrh, Red Raspberry, White Poplar

SPASMS—Convulsions—A sudden, abnormal, involuntary muscular contraction.

see Convulsion, Chorea, Cramps, Cholera, Colic, Epilepsy, Asthma

Bowels—Peppermint, Asafoetida

Croup—Lobelia

Stomach—Asafoetida

Griping—Ginger, Cloves

Weakness—Peruvian Bark

Useful—Cayenne, Asafoetida, Cramp Bark, Pennyroyal, Skullcap, Lobelia, Mistletoe, Wild Yam, Blue Cohosh, Ginger

SPERMATORRHEA—Abnormally frequent involuntary emissions of semen

see Sexual, testicles

Useful—Pipsissewa, Lady's Slipper, False Unicorn, Buchu,
Gravel Root, Asafoetida

Weakness—Cubebs, Skullcap

SPINAL MENINGITIS—*see* Meninges

SPLEEN (Milt)—A highly, vascular or ductless organ situated in
man near the cardiac end of the stomach.

see Blood purifiers

Inflammation (SPLEENITIS)—Vervain, Dandelion

Congested—Culver's Root, American Mandrake, Dandelion,
Senna, Butternut

Useful—Barberry, Dandelion

SPRAIN—*see* Swellings, Bruises

Useful (external applications)—Cayenne, Comfrey, Marshmallow, Lobelia, Hemlock Spruce, Plantain, Mullein, Pennyroyal, Tansy, Figwort

STOMACH—*see* Colic, Gastric, Gastritis, Bilious, Breath, Alvine
Canal, Catarrh

Acidity—*see* Charcoal, Acid, Hiccough

Bleeding—Witch Hazel

Colds—Cayenne, Carrot

Cramp—Bayberry

Canker—Bayberry, Rue

Delicate—Rhubarb

Debilitated—Black Pepper, Cayenne, Carrot, Sage, Red Elm,
Cranesbill, Rhubarb, Golden Seal

Cleans—Vervain, Bayberry, Lobelia, Roman Chamomile,
Barberry, Blessed Thistle

Food not retained—Olive Oil, Red Elm

Hemorrhage—Cranesbill, Beth Rt.

Infantile or children's troubles—Rhubarb, Red Raspberry,
Peppermint

Inflammation—Red Elm, Chickweed

Irritation in Cholera—Purple Loosestrife

Irritated—Eur. Columbo

Lax conditions—White Poplar

Lubricant—Olive Oil

Mucus and mucous membrane—Buchu, Yarrow, Hyssop

Malnutrition—Olive Oil

Narcotic poisoning—Bayberry, Coffee

Nervous—Golden Seal, Roman Chamomile

Pains—Cayenne, Bayberry

Pyloris, inflamed or ulcerated—Red Elm

During pregnancy—False and True Unicorn

Soothing—Peppermint

Sour—Black Horehound, *see* Acid, Charcoal

Sore—Comfrey

Stimulates—Aloes, Prickly Ash

Spasms—Asafoetida

Spasmodic pains—Peppermint

Tonic—Balmony, Pipsissewa, White Horehound, False Unicorn, Cranesbill, Golden Seal, Eur. Gentian, Amer. Centaury, Pleurisy Rt.

Torpid—Horseradish, Cascara Sagrada; *see* Constipation

Ulcers—Red Elm, Sanicle

Useful—Amer. and Eur. Columbo, Red Elm, Yellow Parilla, Cascara Sagrada, Horseradish, Roman Chamomile, White Oak, Amer. Gentian, Bl. Pepper

Quiet after vomiting—Spearmint

Weak and debilitated—Golden Seal, Blessed Thistle

Worms—Santonica, Garlic, False Unicorn, Balmony, Pumpkin seeds

Weak—Eur. Gentian, Eur. Columbo, Red Raspberry, Red Elm, Black Horehound

Warms—Prickly Ash, Ginger, Myrrh, Horseradish, Pennyroyal

see Nausea and vomiting

Digestive weakness in lax conditions—White Poplar, Eur. Gentian

Sluggish with biliousness and torpid bowels—W. Poplar

Irritable nervous depression—Lady's Slipper

STONES or GRAVEL—A calculous concretion in the body, esp. in the kidneys, bladder, or gallbladder.

see Gravel, Kidneys, Bladder, Urinary Organs, Urine, Gall Bladder, Liver, Bilious conditions

The author's method of treating her gall stones is as follows: Once a month, or when distressed, take 1 T. of pure olive oil in 2 T. unsweetened grapefruit juice, 3 nights in a row before retiring. Retire at once and lie on your back or the right side. Do not eat for four hours before taking.

If, during the day, you experience gall stone colic, lie down and take 1 t. pure olive oil every ½ hr. I usually have relief in 1½ hrs. A heating pad at the back helps.

I also take plenty of garlic and parsley capsules. These I take whenever I have the slightest stomach distress.

"Breaker"—Parsley
Useful for stone or gravel—Parsley, Marshmallow, Uva Ursi, Clivers, Bitter Rt., Red Elm, Pipsissewa, Linseed, Hops, Olive Oil, Roman Chamomile
Relieves pain and soothes nerves in gall stones—Wild Yam
Prevent and dissolve—Dandelion
Prevents formation—Uva Ursi

STRANGURIA—Urine emitted with great difficulty and pain, drop by drop.
see Dysuria
Useful—Linseed, Marshmallow
Increases Urine—White Poplar, Uva, Ursi, Marshmallow

SUNBURN—Inflammation of the skin caused by exposure to the sun's rays.
Useful—Aloes
Face—wash with cucumbers

SUNSTROKE—Due to the sun's rays or to excessive heat, marked by sudden prostration, with or without fever.
see Heat, Exhaustion
Specific for exhaustion from overheat—Pennyroyal
Specific for sunstroke—Pennyroyal

SWELLINGS—*see* organ involved, Sprains, Glands
Congested—Sassafras
Bony and Cartilaginous—Poke
Glandular, vicious and severe—Mullein
Scrofulous—Plantain, Mullein
Useful—Marshmallow, Wood Sage, Hops, Mullein, Comfrey, Roman Chamomile, Figwort, Wild Meadow Sage
White averted—Poke

SYPHILIS—A chronic, infectious venereal disease, communicated by contact or heredity, usually has 3 stages: the first (primary syphilis) in which a hard chancre forms at the point of inoculation; the second (secondary syphilis), characterized by skin affections and constitutional disturbances; and the third (tertiary syphilis), characterized by affections of the bone, muscles, viscera, etc.

see Venereal, Chancres

Blood impurities—See Blood Purifiers

Hepatic apparata sluggish—Bitter Rt.

Secondary—Guaiacum, Blue Flag, Yellow Parilla, Queen's Delight, Jam Sarsaparilla

Sores—Golden Seal, White Poplar

Ulcers—Golden Seal

Ulcers, bad Labial (Lips)—Golden Seal

Useful—Bitter Rt., Oregon Grape, Pipsissewa, Black Cohosh, Blue Flag, Queen's Delight, Yellow Parilla, Sassafras

TATTOO—to remove use Nut Galls

TEETH—*see* Gums, Toothache, Breath

Bleeding from extraction—Cranesbill

Clenched—*see* Nerves

Harden gums prior to fitting false—White Oak

Dentifrice—Myrrh

Loose teeth fastened—Pomegranate

TESTICLES—One of the (usually) 2 glands in the male which secrete the spermatozoa, and some of the fluid elements of the semen: (testes).

see Spermatorrhea

Swollen—Chickweed

Inflammation (Orchitis)—*see* Mumps

TETANUS—An infectious, often fatal disease characterized by more or less violent spasms and rigidity of many or all the voluntary muscles, esp. those of the neck and lower jaw (lockjaw).

see Nerves

Useful—Cramp Bark, Lobelia

TETTERS—Any of the various cutaneous diseases

see Eczema, Impetigo, Shingles, Skin, Hands

Useful—White Oak, Sanicle, Elecampane, Red Elm, Plantain

THROAT—*see* Quinsy, Voice, Diphtheria, Adenoids, Tonsils, Hoarseness

Canker—Red Raspberry

Cleanse of Mucus—Sanicle

Infants—Spray with Myrrh

Inflamed and irritated—White Oak, Serpentaria, Cayenne, Myrrh, Cranesbill, Sumach, W. Pond Lily, Thyme

Relaxed—sore—Cayenne, Myrrh, Tormentil, Sage

Sore from cold—Vinegar, Lemon, Pineapple

Sore from croup—Red Elm, Pineapple

Sore from catarrh in Diphtheria—Red Elm

Sore Putrid (foul)—W. Pond Lily, Bayberry, Pineapple

Aphthous ulceration—Cranesbill

Ulcerated—White Oak, Sage, Myrrh, Sanicle, Cayenne, Sumach, Pomegranate

Malignant sore—Cayenne, Serpentaria

Sore and irritated—Golden Seal, Cayenne, Sumach, Red Raspberry, Sage, Queen's Delight, Ginger, Serpentaria, Hyssop, Sanicle, Red Elm, W. Pond Lily, Pomegranate, Purple Loosestrife, Bayberry, Maidenhair, Thyme, Licorice Mullein

Gargle—Cayenne, Barberry

THROMBOSIS—A coagulation of the blood in a bloodvessel or in the heart—*see* Blood Purifiers

THRUSH (Aphthous)—Esp. in children, characterized by whitish spots and ulcers on the membranes of the mouth, fauces, etc., due to a parasitic fungus; often caused by derangement of the stomach; Frog; White Mouth.

see White Mouth, Fauces

Useful—Red Beet

Infants—Rue, White Pond Lily

Useful—G Rue, Myrrh, Plantain

Clean tongue with borax and honey

THYROID—Pertaining to a ductless gland adjacent to the larynx and upper trachea and furnishing an important secretion—known in men as Adam's Apple.

see Goitre, Glands

Goitre (big neck)—Poke

TOADSKIN–(PHRYNODERMA) Useful–Vit. A, Cod Liver Oil

TOBACCO
  Pulmonary troubles–Coltsfoot
  Substitute–Coltsfoot, Lobelia, Cubebs

TONGUE
  Black (low septic conditions)–Echinacea
  Canker–Red Raspberry
  Foul–Boneset
  Paralysis–Ginger
  Ulcers–Myrrh
  Thrush–clean with borax and honey

TONIC–*see* Convalescence, Debility, Dysuria, Digestion, Fevers,
    Organs involved
  Useful–Yarrow, Lady's Slipper, Hops, Golden Seal, Peruvian
    Bark, White Poplar, Eur. Gentian, Amer. Centaury, True
    Unicorn, Bayberry, Roman Chamomile
  Circulation–Myrrh
  Digestive organs–Uva Ursi, Barberry, Eur. Gentian, Yarrow
  Dyspepsia–False Unicorn, Wahoo

TONSILS–see Quinsy, Throat
  Swollen–Hollyhock
  Tonsilitis–Pleurisy Rt., Red Sage

TOOTHACHE–(ODONTALGIA)–*see* Teeth, Gums
  Toothache–Cloves, Prickly Ash, Sassafras, Roman Cham-
    omile, Hops

TRACHOMA–A contagious inflammation of the conjunctiva of
    the eyelids, characterized by the formation of granulations
    or papillary growths.
    see Eyes, Conjunctiva
  Tubercular–Oregon Grape Rt.

TUBERCULOSIS (Consumption)–Progressive wasting of the
    body, esp. from tuberculosis of the lung.
    see Phthisis, Scrofula, Pulmonary troubles
  Cachexy in progressive–Dandelion
  Of the Bowels–Irish Moss
  Difficult and excessive expectoration–Myrrh, Yellow Parilla
  Prevented–Bayberry

Useful—Elecampane and Echinacea combined
Lung—Comfrey, Elecampane, Yellow Parilla, Black Cohosh,
Roman Chamomile
Nutritious—Cod Liver Oil, Chickweed, Red Elm
Nervous—Wild Cherry
Incipient stage of consumption—Charcoal
Trachoma—Oregon Grape Rt.
Pulmonary—Skunk Cabbage, Iceland Moss, Beth Rt. Sanicle,
Eur. Colombo, Asafoetida
Useful—Irish Moss, Red Elm, Echinacea, Polypody, Lobelia,
Wild Cherry, Myrrh, Coltsfoot, Pleurisy Rt., Comfrey,
Bl. Horehound, Mullein, Sanicle
Reduce pulse in paroxysms—Black Cohosh
Paroxysms (convulsive cough)—Black Cohosh
Hectic fever—Wild Cherry

TUMOR—An abnormal or morbid swelling or protuberance in
any part of the body, esp. morbid growth of new tissue not
due to inflammation and differing in structure from the
part in which it grows.
see Growths
Inflamed—White Pond Lily, Red Elm
Painful—Figwort
Useful—Plantain, Chickweed, Pipsissewa, Ground ivy
see Blood Purifiers—Pipsissewa

TYPHOID—Resembling Typhus. An infectious, often fatal febrile
disease, characterized by intestinal inflammation and ulcer-
ation, due to a specific bacillus which is usually introduced
with food or drink.
see Fevers, Typhus
Bowels—Asafoetida
With air in the bowels—Asafoetida
Brain irritation relieved—Lady's Slipper
Arterial excitement relieved—Yarrow
Delirium relieved—Lady's Slipper, Skullcap
Diarrhea—Amer. Colombo
Fecal accumulation—Rhubarb
Excessive discharges, fecal or sanious—Cranesbill
Gangrenous stage—Peruvian Bark
Liver not active enough—Culvers Rt.

Prevented—Boneset
Suppurative—Peruvian Bark
Tonic in convalescence—Amer. Columbo
Useful—Marshmallow, Pleurisy Rt., Cayenne, Boneset, Burdock, Pipsissewa, Lady's Slipper, Gravel Rt., Juniper, Culvers Rt., Lobelia, Serpentaria, Yarrow, Purple Loosestrife, Peruvian Bark, Echinacea, Ginger
If scaling—Red Elm

TYPHUS—An acute infectious disease characterized by great prostration, severe nervous symptoms, and a peculiar eruption of reddish spots on the body: jail-fever, ship-fever; believed to be transmitted through the agency of fleas.
see Typhoid, Fever
Low state—Lady's Slipper
Liver not active enough—Culvers Rt.
Typhus Gravior—Peruvian Bark
Useful—Pleurisy Rt., Lobelia, Serpentaria

ULCERS—A sore open, either to the surface of the body or to a natural cavity, and accompanied by the disintegration of tissue and the formation of pus.
see Organs involved, Canker, Dysentery
Aphthous, see Mouth—Cranesbill
Arrests decomposition (putrification) and deodorized— Charcoal
Dressing after cleansing—Honey
Cornea of the eye—Golden Seal
Gangrenous—Carrot
Indolent—Yellow Parilla, Red Clover, Cranesbill, Chickweed, Prickly Ash, Wood Sage
Obstinate—Comfrey, Pipsissewa
Labial (Lips)—Golden Seal
Varicosed Vein—Sassafrass
Scrofulous—Bayberry
Old—Clivers
Odor, offensive—Charcoal
Sloughing—Eur. Gentian, Carrot
Syphilitic—Golden Seal
Stomach specific—Red Elm
Useful—Hemlock Spruce, Myrrh, Poke, Queen's Delight, Red

Elm, Bayberry, Carrot, Purple Loosestrife, W. Oak, W. Pond Lily, Golden Seal, Ro. Chamomile, Iceland Moss, Sanicle, Red Raspberry, Pipsissewa, Sassafras, Balm of Gilead, Figwort, Linseed

URETHRA—A complete tube extending from the bladder and serving to convey and discharge urine (and, in the male, semen also).

see Urine, Bladder, Gleet, Gonorrhea

Inflamed mucous membrane—Cubebs

Irritation—Buchu, Gravel Rt., Clivers

Irritation, morbid—Buchu

Soothes—Watermelon, Witch Hazel

Useful—Maidenhair, False Unicorn, Watermelon

Inflamed (Urethritis)—Marshmallow, Blue Cohosh

URINARY ORGANS and TRACT—*see* Stones, Bladder

Aged helped—Bayberry

Congested—Uva Ursi

Cleans discharge—Cubebs

Hemorrhage—Marshmallow

Inflamed and irritable—Linseed, Red Elm, Gravel Rt., Licorice.

Mucous membrane—Gravel Root, Uva Ursi, Cubebs, Plantain, Linseed

Obstructions—Clivers, Dandelion

Stricture (Morbid contraction of passage or duct)—Carrots, White Poplar, Uva Ursi

Tonics—White Poplar, Golden Seal, Uva Ursi

Useful—Marshmallow, Uva Ursi, Buchu, Cubebs, Maiden Hair, Hollyhock, Pipsissewa, Guaiacum, Red Elm

Ulcerated—Uva Ursi

URINE—*see* Dysuria, Kidneys, Bright's Disease, Albuminaria, Bladder, Dropsy, Diabetes, Urether, Stones

Bloody—(HEMATURIA)—Sumach, Gravel Rt., Comfrey

Cleans circulation of Urea—Corn Silk

Color red—Rhubarb

Eliminated urates (a salt of Uric Acid)—Buchu

Eliminated solids—Gravel Rt.

Increases flow—Buchu, Parsley, Pipsissewa, Horseradish, Catnip, Gravel Rt., Figwort, Juniper, Corn Silk, Wood Sage,

Burdock, Plantain, White Poplar, Clivers, Uva Ursi, Cubebs

Irritation—Blue Cohosh

Incontinence (unable to retain) in youth and aged—(Enuresis)—Yarrow, W. Poplar, Cranesbill, Uva Ursi, Buchu, Peruvian Bark, Bistort, False Unicorn

Incontinence caused by worms—Santonica

Painful, difficult micturition (desire to morbidly frequent)—Gravel Rt.

Mucous in—Buchu, Burdock

Prevents too frequent—Blue Cohosh

Purulent decomposition in—Corn Silk

Obstructions—Pipsissewa, Carrots

Relieves strong odor of Ammonia—Corn Silk

Relieves strong odor—Charcoal

Retention (suppression)—Juniper, Spearmint, Carrot, Uva Ursi, Buchu, Clivers

Scanty in fevers, with or without brick dust deposits—Gravel Rt.

Scrofula—urine flow increased—Poke

Sugar—*see* Diabetes

Scalding—Burdock, Maiden Hair, Clivers, Plantain, Red Elm, Cubebs, Gravel Rt.

Increase in Stranguria—W. Poplar, Uva Ursi, Marshmallow

Useful—Corn Silk

Weakness in aged—Buchu

Back ache in incontinence—White Poplar

Uric Acid—Juniper, Buchu

Yellow—Satonica

PROLAPSED UTERI—Falling down of the uterus (womb)—*see* Uterus

Useful—Uva Ursi, False Unicorn, Amer. Columbo, Witch Hazel, Bayberry, White Pond Lily, White Oak, Beth Rt., Sumac

UTERUS—(Womb)

see Prolapsus Uteri, Cervix, Menstruation, Partuition, Generative organs, Hemorrhage

Atony—False Unicorn, Juniper

Atony with constipation and flatulence—Aloes

Barrenness—False and True Unicorn, Catnip

Cramps during pregnancy—Wild Yam

Cleans mucous membrane—Bl. Horehound, Motherwort

Congested—Roman Chamomile

Flaccid (limp)—Uva Ursi

Fibroids—Blue Flag

Hyperaemia (excessive accumulation of blood)—Wild Yam

Irritated and inflamed—Blue Cohosh, Lady's Slipper, Gravel Rt., Red Elm

Pains—Wild Yam

Relaxant—Cramp Bark

Rheumatism—Black Cohosh, Cramp Bark

Os Uteri, (Orifice of the Uterus) rigid—Lady's Slipper, Lobelia, Blue Cohosh

Sluggish—Juniper

Stimulant—Aloes

Tonic—G. Rue, Red Raspberry, False and True Unicorn, Myrrh, Witch Hazel

Tonic in Pregnancy—False Unicorn

Ulcers—Amer. Columbo, Golden Seal

Useful—Maiden Hair, Ro. Chamomile, Black Cohosh, Bayberry, False Unicorn Rt., Gravel Rt., Serpentaria, Amer. Columbo

Weakness—Red Elm, White Poplar, Pipsissewa

UVULA—A small, fleshy, conical body projecting downward from the middle of the soft palate.

Relaxed or elongated—Ginger, Cayenne, Sage, Hollyhock, Cranesbill

Prolapsed—White Oak

VAGINA—The passage leading from the uterus to the vulva in a female.

see Vulva, Leucorrhea, Gonorrhea

Catarrh—Witch Hazel

Flaccid (limp)—Uva Ursi

Relaxed—Witch Hazel, White Oak, False Unicorn, White Pond Lily

Stimulating—Aloes

Tonic—Witch Hazel

Ulcers—Amer. Columbo, Golden Seal

Vaginitis (irritated and inflamed)—Blue Cohosh, Red Elm, Gravel Rt., Motherwort
Wash (Douche)—Marshmallow, White Pond Lily
Weak—Pipsissewa, Amer. Columbo, Beth Rt., White Poplar
Laxity—Yarrow

VEINS—*see* Arteries, Lymphatics
Varicose—Witch Hazel
Varicose Ulcers—Sassafras
Prominent—Witch Hazel
Red—Witch Hazel

VENEREAL DISEASES—Arising from sexual intercourse with an infected person.
see Gonorrhea, Syphilis, Chancre
Rheumatism—Guaiacum
Useful—Blue Flag, Burdock

VERTIGO—Dizziness, giddiness; a disordered state, as of the mind—*see* Dizziness

VOICE—*see* Throat, Laryngitis, Hoarseness
Gargle—Cayenne, Sage
Congestion in vocal cords—White Horehound

VOMITING—*see* Nausea, Cholera, Pregnancy
Allays—Cloves, Peppermint, Wild Yam, Spearmint, Charcoal
Quiets stomach after—Spearmint

VULVA—The external genital organs of the female; esp. the orifice of these.
see Vagina, Chancre
Excoriations—White Pond Lily
Irritable chancres—White Pond Lily
Pruritis (Itching)—Tansy

WARTS—*see* Growths
Remove—Wild Meadow Sage, Castor Oil

WHITLOWS—An inflammation of the deeper tissues of a finger or toe, esp. of the terminal phalanx, usually terminating in suppuration.
see Felon, Feet
Slip the finger into a hole cut into a lemon.

WORMS—(Taenia)

Tonic to bowels after expelling worms—Yarrow

In children—Balmony, Amer. Wormseed, Butternut

In Intestines—Amer. Wormseed

In Stomach—Santonica, Garlic, False Unicorn, Balmony

Seat—Santonica

Pin Worms—Pomegranate, Aloes, Santonica

Round Worms—Santonica, Pomegranate

Tape specific—Pomegranate

Tape—Male Fern, Pomegranate, Tansy, Polypody, Butternut, Santonica, Pumpkin Seeds

Thread—Tansy

Useful—Bitter Rt., Eur. Gentian, Tansy, G. Rue, Aloes, Vervain, Hyssop, Hops, Santonica, Male Fern, Pumpkin Seeds

Incontinence of urine caused by worms—Santonica

YELLOW FEVER—A dangerous, often fatal, infectious febrile disease of warm climates, transmitted by the bite of a mosquito, and characterized by jaundice, vomiting, and hemorrhages.

see Fevers

Useful—Cayenne, Boneset

INDEX

234

About the Author

Henrietta A. Diers Rau has led a long and busy life. Born in Bremen, Germany, Mrs. Rau became a naturalized citizen of the United States in 1922. She took secretarial courses at Egan's Business School in Hoboken, N.J., and accounting with the La Salle Extension University. She was an office manager for several years until she became interested in real estate. She then studied real estate at Caldwell Institute in Orange, N.J., real estate law at the City College of New York, business economics at Rutgers University of Newark, N.J., and insurance at the Aetna Insurance Company in Hartford, N.J. For twenty-five years she had her own real estate and insurance business in Rahway, N.J., retiring to take care of her mother and sister when they became ill with cancer. It was at this point Mrs. Rau began to study medical herbs in earnest.

In 1955, she received the degree of Master Herbalist from Dominion Herbal College in Vancouver, British Columbia, Canada. Then she took a three-year course in medical herbs at the National Association of Medical Herbalists of Great Britain, Ltd. Finally, in 1964, she received her diploma of Naturopathy after writing a medical thesis for the Anglo-American Institute of Drugless Therapy of Great Britain.

A resident of Rahway, N.J., Mrs. Rau is a frequent lecturer on herbs and herbal medicines and has published articles in *Organic Gardening and Farming*, the *Elizabeth Daily Journal*, *Women's Circle*, and *Cosmos*.